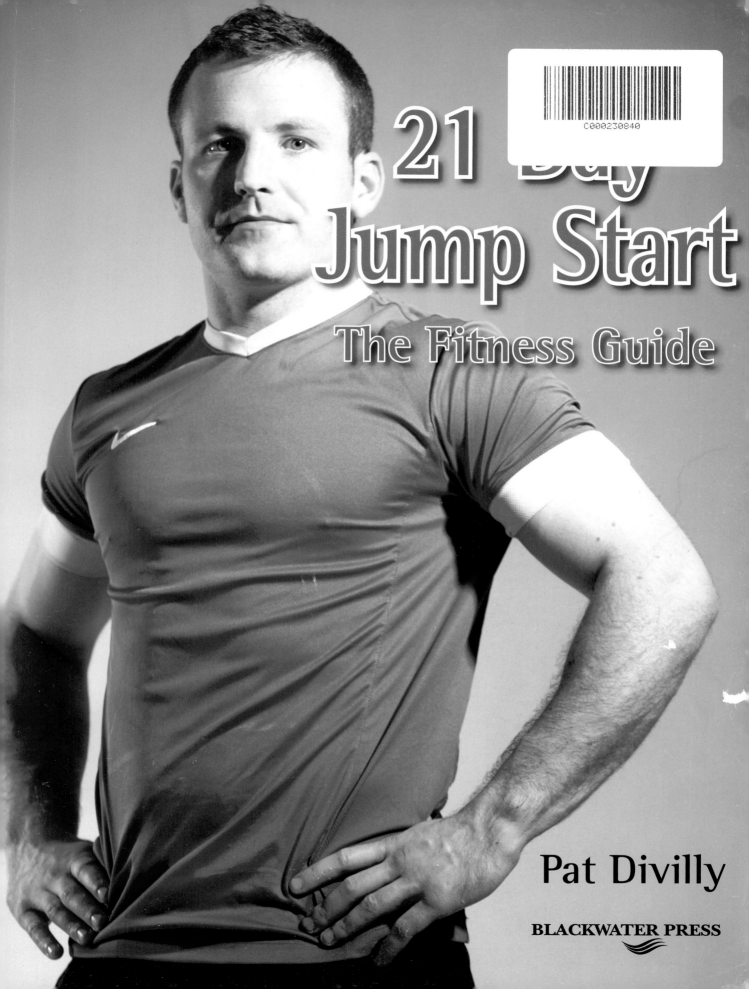

21 Day Jump Start
The Fitness Guide

Pat Divilly

BLACKWATER PRESS

ISBN 978-0-9576170-7-0

BWP Ltd., 1-5 North Frederick Street, Dublin 1
Printed in the Republic of Ireland.

jloconnor@eircom.net

Layout and Design: Artwerk Limited

Contents

DEDICATION

I'd like to dedicate this book to my parents.
Thank you for your constant support, encouragement and love.

Acknowledgements

I would like to thank my publisher John O'Connor for giving me the opportunity to publish this book and all the team at Blackwater Press for their help in getting it over the line.

I would like to thank all my clients who agreed to be featured in this book for their testimonials. I would also like to thank Evan Doherty for the photography and Tara King for all her ideas and advice while writing the manuscript.

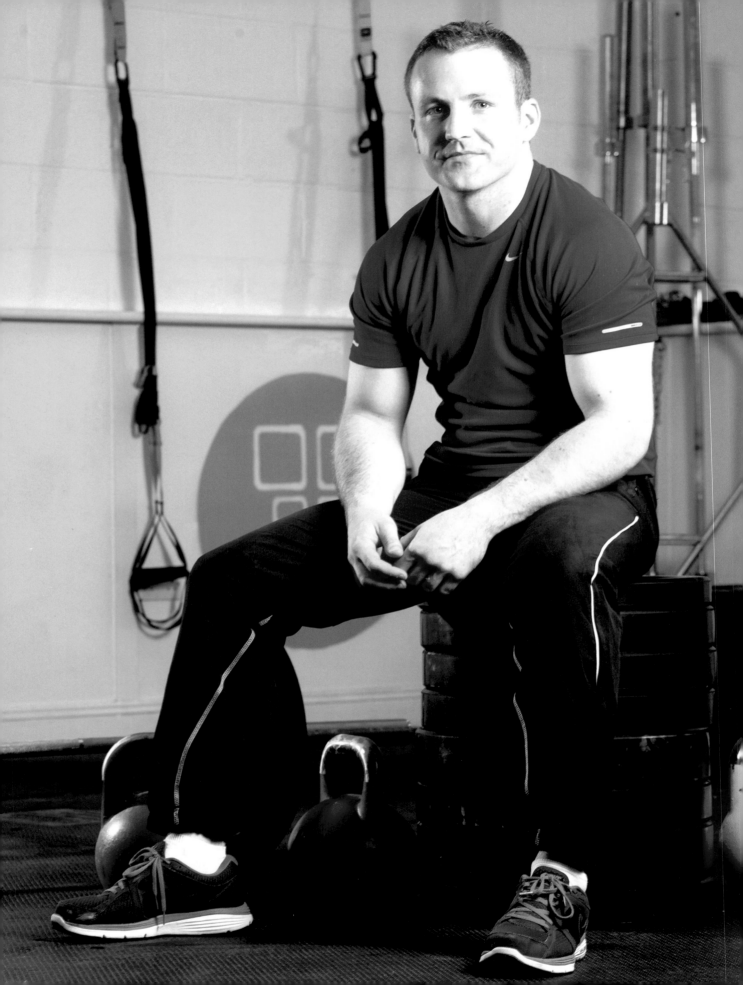

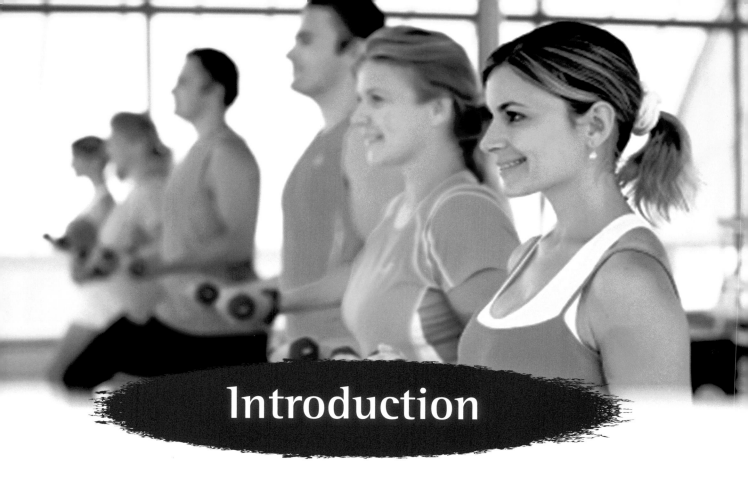

Introduction

As a personal trainer based in Galway and having had huge success with my clients on their fitness and weight loss journeys since I founded Pat Divilly Fitness in 2011, I wrote this book as a guide for the everyday person who is looking to feel, look and move better.

There is so much information out there with regard to training and nutrition but the scale of it leaves people feeling confused and overwhelmed. What you will find in *21 Day Jump Start* is concise information that's action-orientated and easy to follow. With a combination of advice, exercise, recipes and a plan of action for each of your 21 days, it will help you achieve results quickly and sustainably.

I've been lucky enough to learn from some of the best nutritionists, trainers and strength coaches in the world and in *21 Day Jump Start* I make this knowledge readily available to anyone who is ready to make a change in their lives. Whatever your weight or level of fitness, if you commit to this plan, you will see results.

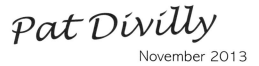

Pat Divilly

November 2013

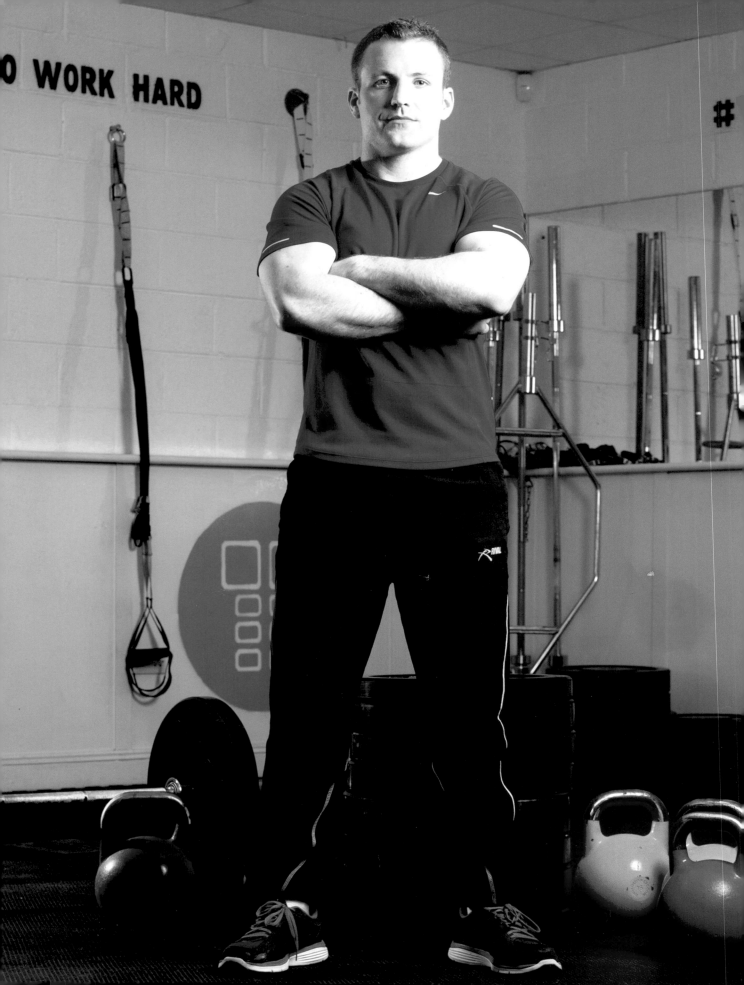

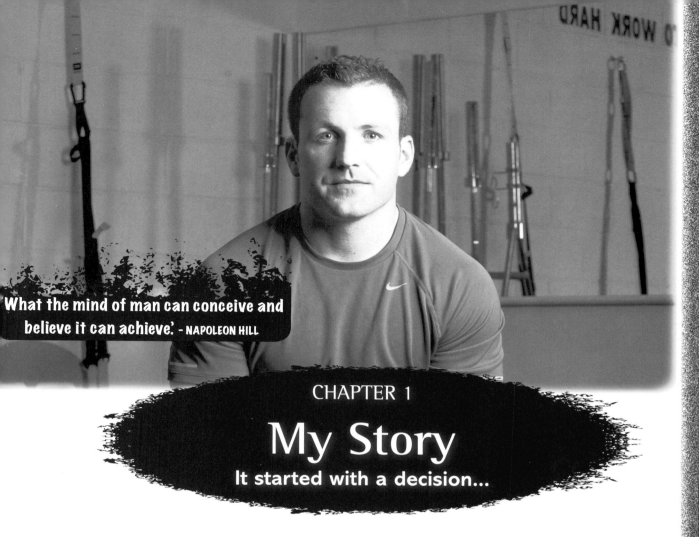

CHAPTER 1

My Story

It started with a decision...

Judo and rugby first brought me to the gym in my early teens and from the day I started I knew what I wanted to do with my life. I began my personal training career whilst completing a Masters in Exercise and Nutrition Science at the University of Chester in England. Working 30 hours per week in the university gym and studying full time, I became completely immersed in all things training and nutrition. Upon completion of my Masters, I moved back to Ireland and began work at a gym in Dublin before setting up as a freelance trainer. Though some of my clients saw fantastic results by following the guidelines I had learnt during my formal studies, others saw little or no change despite following my training and nutrition recommendations to the letter. This frustrated me and left me a little disillusioned, wondering whether I had a future in personal training. With few contacts in the big city and having started my business at such a young age I had a hard time standing out from the legions of trainers in Dublin.

Determined to make it work and keep the dream alive, I got some part-time work in a clothes shop to help pay the bills, but after months of struggling to pay the rent and stay afloat I was forced to move home to Galway to live with my parents at twenty-four years of age. I got the bus from Dublin at 2pm on Christmas Eve 2011 after finishing my shift at the clothes shop. I'll never forget my dad having to send me money for my bus fare or having to borrow money to buy my mum a Christmas present that year. Worse again with her birthday being on Christmas Day. I could only provide a card promising 'lunch in the new year' – a card that might as well have said that despite all the opportunities my parents had given me I was twenty-four and had nothing to show for myself. I had hit an all-time low and wasn't sure where to go next.

I got some part-time work in a restaurant in Galway and weighed up my options. Physiotherapy would provide me with more security and still allow me to help people feel and move better. When I got a place on a physiotherapy course in England, I seemed to have found the light at the end of the tunnel, but I was quickly knocked back days later when I was informed that the NHS were no longer funding the course and that there weren't any places available.

I struggled with anxiety and sleepless nights, before eventually making a decision. Fitness and health had been my passion since my early teens. I remember setting foot in the gym for the first time and promising myself that someday I'd have my own gym. Other trainers were making a good living helping people to change their lives. Why couldn't I do the same? Things hadn't worked out for me in Dublin but I reminded myself that 'your failures do not define you'. Determined to make it work I began seeking out the trainers who were getting the best results. I sent emails asking for book recommendations, advice and ideas. I immersed myself in studying anything that would help me get better results for potential clients.

While still working in the restaurant, I began training friends for free to test out everything I was learning. I had found purpose again. Every waking minute was dedicated to learning. When I wasn't working in the restaurant, I was reading, watching videos or attending seminars. I took the little bit of money I had saved and had 5,000 flyers printed advertising a fitness camp at the local beach. With work being so hard to come by because of the recession I took a chance by leaving my job at the restaurant to pursue the 'dream'. I was going to make this work...

I ran my first fitness camp on the beach in Barna, my hometown in the west of Ireland, with a handful of clients. I wasn't driving, so instead I would get up at 6am most mornings and cycle to the beach for 7am, then again at 9.45am and again in the evening. Despite the early mornings, cycling and training in the rain, and the long days, I was happier than I'd been in months. I invested my earnings from the fitness camps in more courses, books and seminars. I travelled all over Europe to learn from strength coaches, nutritionists, microbiologists, psychologists and anyone else who was helping people to get healthier.

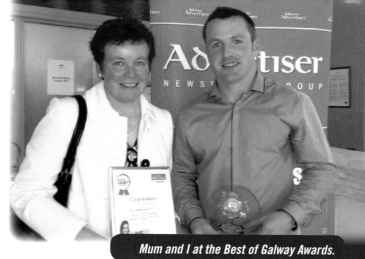

Mum and I at the Best of Galway Awards.

Word soon began to spread about the results my clients were getting and my camps began to grow. My confidence in getting results using everything I'd learned about health and fitness techniques over the previous months allowed me to offer a 200% money back guarantee on my classes. By October 2012, I was training upwards of 100 people a day at the beach – wind, rain or shine. Word had spread beyond Galway and I started getting requests from people across the country and abroad looking for training and nutrition plans. My motivation only grew with each testimonial I received from clients reporting improvements not only to their health and wellness but to their personal and business lives.

December brought another victory when I was able to buy my mum the Christmas and birthday presents she deserved. A few months later, I was able to take her out for that lunch to the 'Best of Galway' awards, where my business was announced as the publicly chosen winner of the category, 'Best In Health/Beauty'.

This past May, less than a year to the day since I started my camps on the beach in Barna, I realised my dream and opened my first studio a few hundred metres from my family home.

I now train clients at my studio in Barna, but I also train hundreds of clients worldwide each month via my online programmes. I continue to travel and learn from some of the best coaches in the world and I have made it my goal to make everything I have

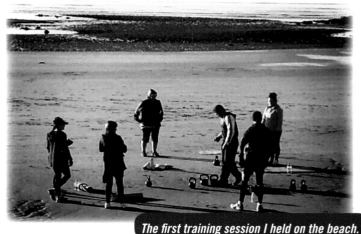

The first training session I held on the beach.

learned readily available to anyone who genuinely wants to improve the way they look, move, and feel.

My *21 Day Jump Start* is a practical, action-orientated programme designed to help you quickly regain your health and vitality. It is an accumulation of information I have picked up from men and women much smarter than I, but, I am proud to share it, as I genuinely believe this guide has the potential to help you change your fitness and your life if you commit to adopting its principles and making them a part of your life. I have shared my story in the hope that it inspires you to live life on your own terms and go after what you want. I believe you picked up this book because you would like to be a happier, healthier version of your current self. I am going to give you all the tools you need. You just need to make the decision!

I am still learning all the time, and no doubt my approach to nutrition and training will change over time – 'only a fool never changes his mind!' – but, I am confident the information and game plan laid out in this book will lead to incredible improvements in the health, wellbeing and happiness of anyone who puts it into action. Hearing the success stories of my clients is just one of the highlights of my job as a health professional, and I look forward to meeting you, the reader, some day and hearing your success story.

Allow yourself 21 days to follow this plan to the letter, and I promise it will jump start your journey toward weight loss, long term weight control, and life long health.

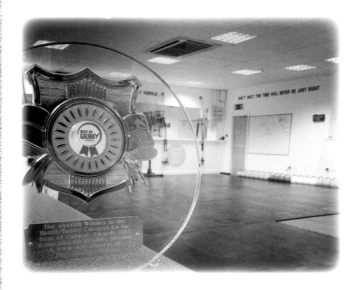

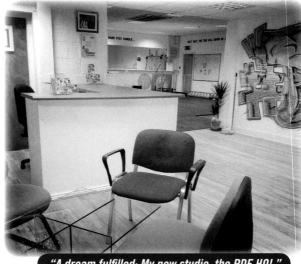

"A dream fulfilled: My new studio, the PDF HQ! "

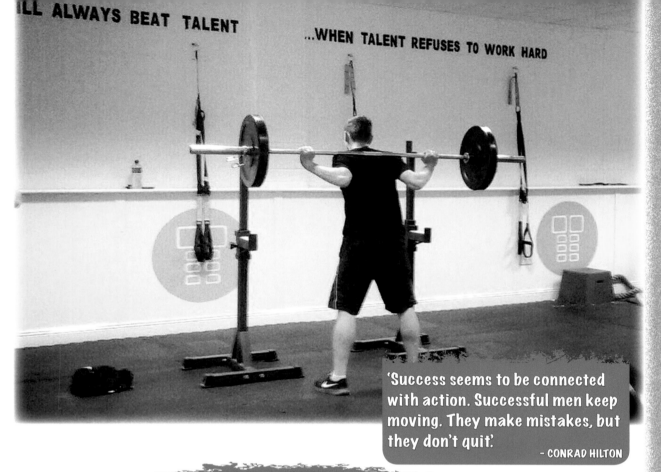

ILL ALWAYS BEAT TALENT

...WHEN TALENT REFUSES TO WORK HARD

'Success seems to be connected with action. Successful men keep moving. They make mistakes, but they don't quit'.
— CONRAD HILTON

CHAPTER 2

Don't Wait – The Time Will Never be Just Right!

I would be willing to bet that this isn't the first diet or training book you've bought. In fact, if you are anything like most you probably already own quite a few. I've heard it said that nowadays we are 'thirsty for knowledge but drowning in information'. With the prominence of the internet and media there have never been so many resources so readily available to us, particularly in the areas of training, nutrition and health. Having access to so much information, research, and studies should make pursuing better health straight forward, but, in reality, it often leaves people feeling confused and overwhelmed.

Many of us become guilty of 'paralysis by analysis'. We become obsessed with reading and talking about the latest diet or fitness trends. We'll spend money each and every month in pursuit of the 'secret' or the 'magic pill'. We'll spend hours trawling the internet reading about different approaches to diet and exercise. But only days into a new training programme we will become distracted by an article outlining a celebrity's training plan and we'll hop on to that instead. Less than a week into a new 'diet' we'll see an advertisement for new slimming pills and feel the need to add them to our plan. Next we'll feel obliged to switch to another plan after seeing the results one of our work colleagues is getting with their new approach to training.

It's a cycle of jumping from one programme or 'magic pill' to another without ever finding a solution that is enjoyable, results-driven and most importantly sustainable. Does this sound familiar? I ask that for the next 21 days you'll commit to the plan laid out in this book 100%. You will hopefully read the book and have your eyes opened to some new ideas and principles. You may at times read it and think, 'well I already know that'. You might know it but are you doing it? I think we are all guilty of this at times. Everybody is looking for the secret formula to success, but they always look externally for this big secret. The closest thing we've got to a secret formula is internal and it's our ability to take action on what we already know.

> 'Knowing is not enough, we must apply. Willing is not enough, we must do.'
> – BRUCE LEE

The most successful people in life don't get caught up in the small details. They don't spend any more time than necessary planning or plotting. Once they have their plan, they take action on it. With the *21 Day Jump Start* you've got the plan that brings success within your reach. It's up to you to take action! I read a statistic that only around 10% of people who start reading a book actually get to the end! I think that's worth thinking about. Please commit to reading through to the end and making this plan a game changer for you! This can either be another book gathering dust on your bookshelf or it can be the book that truly transforms your health and your life.

My goal is to put you in a position of power. I want you to know why you should be eating certain foods and not others. I want you to know why certain supplements can greatly benefit you and why some forms of exercise are far superior to others. The countless 'diets' sold today do little more than set people up for failure. We should be free to eat and enjoy delicious foods that keep us fit, strong and healthy without having to weigh foods or make calorie counting a part-time profession!

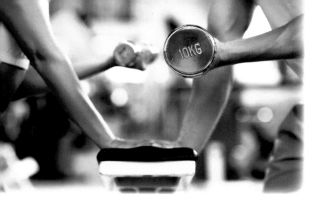

Training should be an enjoyable part of life, not a chore that takes up all of our free time. Instead of 'falling off the wagon' on day 22 or before, I want you to become excited about making the principles in this book a part of your life going forward. This isn't a quick fix solution like the many that have come before. It's an introduction to a new way of living that promotes effortless weight loss, vibrant energy and lifelong health. The principles outlined will involve some changes to what you are currently doing, maybe some big changes, but I won't be asking you to live like a monk or nun!

The media make their money by selling us images of what healthy, lean and sexy are and how we can become these things. But following their guidelines has only left us sick, tired, and out of pocket! Only we can take responsibility for our own health. It isn't in the hands of the media, our doctors, our families or friends. It's up to us to understand what it takes to be healthy and to take the necessary steps to get there. Before we start our jump start toward weight loss and improved health we need to look at why we are here.

How Did We Get Here?

As a nation we're overweight, tired, run down and sick. We're overfed and undernourished. Obesity levels are at an all-time high, stress levels are through the roof and we've become dependent on sugar and caffeine to function normally. Diseases that were practically non-existent in our grandparents' time are rampant now and cases of chronic degenerative diseases are on the rise. Government nutrition guidelines have become outdated and even though as a nation we're training more, following low fat diets and taking weight loss pills and potions, only a small percentage of the population are lean, strong and experiencing the kind of good health we are all supposed to have. We have come to believe that it's standard to need coffee or sugar to wake up in the morning or that it's normal to go to bed at night shattered but jumpy and unable to sleep. We've come to think we 'need' fat burners, low calorie diets and marathon training sessions to lose weight. We've become reliant on medication and drugs to rid us of any physical or mental ailment or condition. We've moved further and further from nature and closer and closer to sickness.

Something has gone terribly wrong.

How We Created A Toxic Environment

Food, stress and sedentary lifestyles have brought us to this point. We all know how quickly technology changes. For most of us it's hard to remember a time before Facebook, mobile phones, hands-free kits, fast food, diet drinks and commercial gyms. We live in a very different age to the generations before us and although we live in an era of convenience and technology we are victims of our evolution and the fast-paced, stress-filled world we have created for ourselves. We now live in a toxic environment where it takes a conscious effort to get healthy and stay healthy.

Remember: being overweight is simply a side effect of being unhealthy so we can thank the toxic environment we have created for the extra 'cushion' we are carrying. There is a clear link between the changes in nutrition over the years and the increase in sickness, disease and obesity. DNA evidence shows that human physiology has not changed over the past 40,000 years. Therefore, our nutritional requirements should, in theory, not be any different to the requirements of our caveman ancestors who lived in the Palaeolithic era which lasted from around 2.5 million years ago to 10,000 years ago. These cavemen and women ate wild meats and seafood, vegetables, nuts, seeds and in season fruits. A select number of indigenous tribes still eating this way show all the signs of exceptional health. Their skin is clear, teeth straight, bodies lean and strong, a far cry from the body of the average Westerner!

The agricultural revolution which came about around 10,000 years ago brought with it some massive changes, bringing grains to the table. Cereals began to make up a bigger part of the typical diet than before and mineral and vitamin deficiencies began to emerge. More recently, in the last 50 years we have seen more change in the way we eat than in the previous 10,000 years. I'll bet a large percentage of the foods at your local supermarket would have been unrecognisable to your grandparents when they were your age! Alongside the increase in consumption of refined sugars and processed foods over the last 50 years we have seen a growing percentage of the population pile on the pounds whilst becoming more and more unhealthy.

We have been told for years now that in order to lose weight we need to burn more calories than we consume. As a result, food producers pump foods full of additives, preservatives and chemicals to mirror the drug-like properties of sugar whilst keeping the calorie count low or non-existent.

With little regard for the quality of the foods being eaten and an obsession with calories in versus calories out, we've sent our bodies into hormonal chaos, making weight loss and overall health impossible.

Stress, an ever-increasing state in our modern world, causes similar hormonal chaos and leads to further weight gain and sickness. To our caveman ancestors the stress or 'fight or flight' response could have meant the difference between life and death. Being perhaps attacked by a lion, the caveman would experience an extremely stressful event which would be over within minutes at which point the stress response would be switched off. Unfortunately for us, our bodies cannot tell the difference between different types of stress.

A typical day might begin with the stress of being suddenly awoken by the alarm clock, followed by the stress of traffic on the way to work, and then the stress of dealing with difficult customers and so on and so forth. It is when this stress response is constantly being switched on and becomes a chronic condition, and not an acute one, that we experience a major decline in health and wellbeing, as well as an increase in body fat accumulation particularly around the stomach area.

Training, which can be another type of stress, can further contribute to the problem. We go to the gym with great intentions but oftentimes only make the situation worse. Chronic cardio, with hours spent in the gym or on the road, can not only tax the joints and muscles but also the body's endocrine system.

In order to drop body fat, improve energy levels and move toward being happier, healthier people we need to eliminate as many of these toxins as we can and create a winning environment where we can thrive and not just survive. The difference we can make in just a few short weeks by making changes to the way we eat, the way we train and the way we manage stress is incredible. Even after months or years of neglect we can quickly turn things around. Your body wants to be lean, strong, fit and healthy. Evolution has taught us the 'secrets' of optimal health but with modern-day living we are moving further and further away from nature.

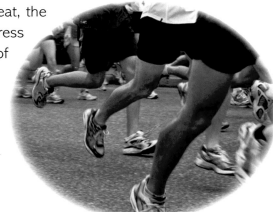

Kim McGoona (Galway)

I have gained so much more from working with Pat than I could have ever anticipated. I started his programme with two things in mind. Weight loss, and knowing I had to give it all I could. I was just so fed up. What I've got in return is a healthier body and mind, an amazing transformation and pride in myself and my abilities. I've experienced endless energy, my skin has cleared up, and best of all... sleep! As a person who has suffered from bouts of insomnia and broken sleep for years, this was paramount for me.

On a daily basis we walk around uncomfortable, bloated, with indigestion, and it's only when you do a programme like Pat's that you realise how you're

Results of Kim's 28 day plan

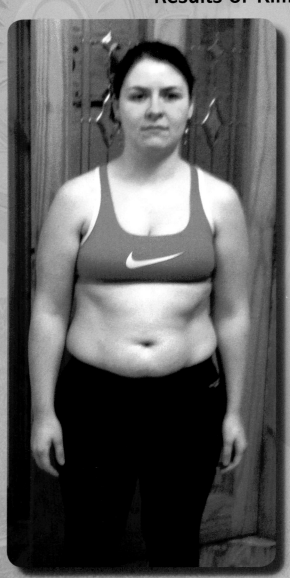
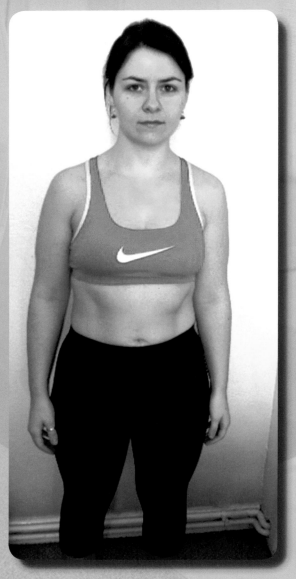

really supposed to feel! I'll never go back. Through this programme, I discovered that I have a dairy intolerance, and now I feel amazing without it in my life. My 'before' and 'after' photos tell a story of weight loss. My friends and family can tell you I'm a different person! I started with 'diet' and 'weight loss' in mind, but I've come away from it a happy, healthier, person who has broken bad habits and made a lifestyle change that is here to stay. I have never felt better and I can only thank Pat for this programme, his guidance, and for helping me find my feet on this.

Results of Kim's 28 day plan

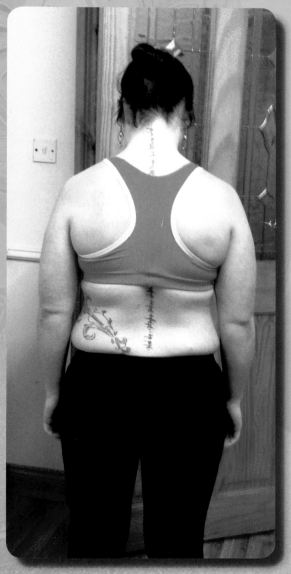
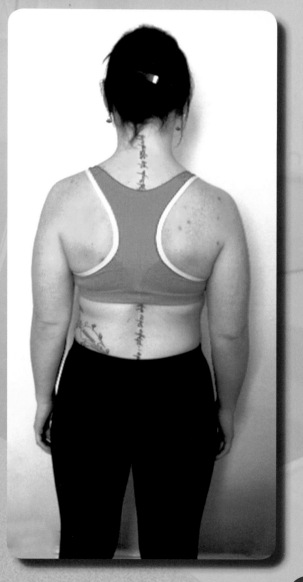

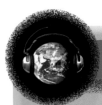

Pat Divilly's Motivational Play List

Here are some of my personal iPod favourites to help keep me going through those tough workouts!

1. Kanye West – Stronger
2. Outkast – B.O.B.
3. Eminem – 8 Mile
4. Jay Z – 99 Problems
5. John O'Callaghan – Find Yourself
6. Oasis – Acquiesce
7. Asap Rocky Skrillex – Wild for the night
8. Foo Fighters – Everlong
9. Lil Wayne and Drake – Right Above It
10. Rage Against The Machine – Bulls on parade
11. Foo Fighters – Best of you
12. Ludacris – Get Back
13. Cypress Hill – Rock Superstar
14. The XX – Intro
15. Hans Zimmer – Time
16. Rusko – Everyday
17. Breaking Benjamin – The Diary Of Jane
18. Roy Jones – Can't be touched
19. Eminem – Till I Collapse
20. Professor Green – Monster (Remix)

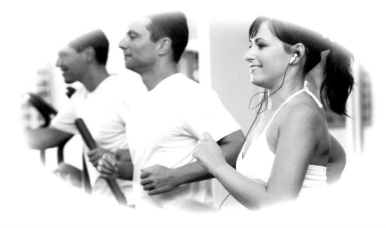

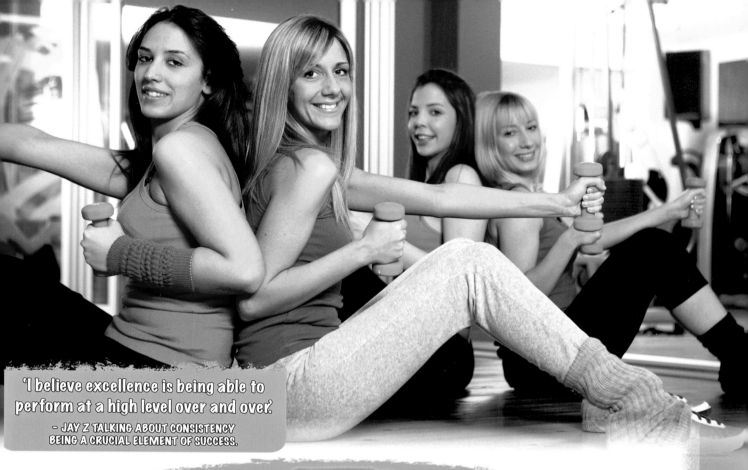

'I believe excellence is being able to perform at a high level over and over'.
– JAY Z TALKING ABOUT CONSISTENCY BEING A CRUCIAL ELEMENT OF SUCCESS.

CHAPTER 3

Envisioning Your Success

Different people are inspired by different things, and this is why it's important that you find the goal-setting strategy that will work best for you.

Everything you do will either take you a step closer or a step further away from your goal, and the more solid a foundation you have, the higher the chance of success. The key is clarity. Don't settle for a vague dream, be as specific as possible. It becomes more achievable that way because you know exactly what you are working towards. If, for instance, you decide you want to set up your own business, then ask yourself every day if your actions are catapulting you closer to your goal or taking you further away from it.

Write down what you want, print these goals in the form of pictures and place them on a vision board. Tell other people about what you intend to do and outline how you intend to put these plans into action. By doing all this, you are building on the strength of the goals and reaffirming them to yourself. It's no longer just a dream, but instead a very real plan!

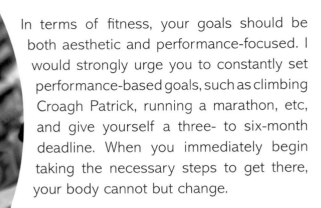

In terms of fitness, your goals should be both aesthetic and performance-focused. I would strongly urge you to constantly set performance-based goals, such as climbing Croagh Patrick, running a marathon, etc, and give yourself a three- to six-month deadline. When you immediately begin taking the necessary steps to get there, your body cannot but change.

Most importantly, stay away from the weighing scales. If you work towards a goal that will improve your performance, then your weight loss and health will take care of themselves. Don't obsess over weight loss. When you are mentally fixated with the weighing scales, the stress will make it impossible to lose weight. As I will explain in greater detail later on, you simply cannot lose weight when your body is stressed.

Your body adapts to the stresses you place on it, be they good or bad forms of stress. Consequently, if you are fixated on losing body fat, then your body is going to respond by holding on to it. It won't perform optimally. If, however, you condition yourself for a specific event or test, then your body will evolve towards that goal. It will adapt accordingly, and that's when you will start to see results.

The Vision Board

Anyone who knows me knows that my favourite book is Napoleon Hill's *Think and Grow Rich*. My dad gave it to me when I was around 15 years of age; I think he was trying to get me focused in time for finishing school. Even though it was written in the 1930s, that book definitely had, and still continues to have, the biggest impact on me. For those who don't know, Napoleon Hill was a writer who famously spent a number of years with the most successful people in the world. He learned their habits, picked up on the various things they would do to be successful, and then outlined his findings in his book.

'I've always considered myself to be just average talent and what I have is a ridiculous insane obsessiveness for practice and preparation.'
– WILL SMITH

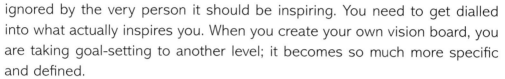

It is so important to surround yourself with anything that will motivate you. I often went through my Dad's bookshelves because they were always filled with inspirational books like Napoleon Hill's. I didn't realise it at the time, but I was actively surrounding myself with success stories. This had a massive influence on me in the years that followed.

When it comes to motivational books and tools, I would strongly recommend that you choose wisely and selectively. A big problem with a lot of them is that they don't focus enough on taking action and working for things. The vision board is a great concept, but it's no good if it just sits on the wall being ignored by the very person it should be inspiring. You need to get dialled into what actually inspires you. When you create your own vision board, you are taking goal-setting to another level; it becomes so much more specific and defined.

I personally love vision boards, and I have been actively using them for the past number of years. I didn't always print the images, but I would most definitely keep them visible on my computer so that I was constantly reminded of what I was working towards. On my vision board right now, there is a picture of a kettlebell certification that I have got coming up, definitely the toughest one I'll have completed yet. There's a picture of Iceland, as my Dad and I have always wanted to travel there. There is also an image of a group of people who have just finished a mud run. I put that particular picture up because I'm bringing my clients to Scotland for a mud run soon and I have a vision of us all enjoying the event and buzzing afterwards. Then there are the pictures relating to this book, such as a signing in Easons, a *Late Late Show* appearance… whatever I envision, I place an image of it on the board!

Your own vision board might be an A3 sheet or a pin-board which you have placed on your bedroom wall or above your desk. It might even just be a few pictures on the fridge door. It doesn't matter what form your vision board takes, the most important thing is to ensure that it is constantly within your line of sight. When you are reminded of your goals on a regular basis, it keeps your motivation from waning.

Don't stick up pictures that are simply nice to look at. Choose only the ones that will inspire and drive you. For body-related goals, maybe put up a picture of the kind of physique you are striving for. Just make sure you have a perfectly clear visual concept of what you want your end result to be.

ENVISIONING YOUR SUCCESS

Reverse Engineering

Reverse engineering is like a GPS for your mind. It solidifies your goals and forces you to outline the various steps you would have to take in order to successfully achieve them.

It doesn't matter if your goal pertains to fitness, finances, relationships or education, reverse engineering is a useful tool that can be applied to whatever it is that you are dreaming of.

You see, your brain works better when it has a defined plan to operate from. This is why reverse engineering is the equivalent of providing a map for your brain. You are outlining to yourself where you want to be, what actions you need to take in order to get there, and the actions you need to change in order to progress.

To begin, write down the end result on an A4 sheet of paper. Where do you want to be? What do you want to feel like? Inject plenty of emotion into your words, and don't use bland language! Be positive and this will help fire up your enthusiasm. When you are detailing your end result, its crucial that you write it in the present tense, as this will reinforce the goal in your subconscious.

For example, you might say:

> 'By September, I weigh ten pounds less than I currently do. I feel stronger than I have ever felt and I enjoy being healthy and strong. I enjoy feeling so energised from eating such healthy foods.'

I can't emphasise enough how important it is to have a clear time frame. A time frame will immediately transform the dream into an attainable goal.

The next most important factor in the reverse engineering process is identifying your 'brakes'. If you have one foot on the accelerator and another on the brake, then the car isn't going to move. The same applies when it comes to your goals. A 'brake' is something that is hindering, or undoing, any productive attempts you are making to move forward. For instance, if you are working towards a 10k race, and you have been 100% committed to your diet and workouts, but you go out drinking each weekend as a treat, then the drink is the 'brake'. If you want to be ten pounds lighter, ask yourself what is stopping you from being ten pounds lighter right now? What are you doing wrong? Maybe you snack on biscuits when the 3pm slump kicks in at work, or maybe you eat too many processed foods late at night? Again, these are 'brakes'.

Once you have identified the 'brakes', outline the necessary actions that you will take to overcome them. Maybe you can still go out at weekends but cut back your alcohol consumption to once a month?

The moment you are clear in your mind about what exactly you want, and what is stopping you from getting it, then you should have no problem achieving your goal.

Here are some questions to help you start your own reverse engineering task:

Outline your perfect picture of health
List the reasons why you are not already in perfect health?
What specific new actions can you take to help you achieve your perfect health?
What is your exact deadline to have this goal achieved by?

Everything comes back to the question 'Why?'. Why do you want this? Why are you doing this? Why are you working towards this? On the days when you are feeling uninspired, look back on your reverse engineering layout, and this will remind you why!

'Everything you do is going to take you a step closer, or a step further away, from your goal.' - PAT DIVILLY

The Compound Effect

The Compound Effect, which was devised by the hugely inspirational Darren Hardy, basically means that small actions, carried out consistently, will lead to a massive result in the end.

Maybe you don't want to make massive changes, so how about making a series of small changes on a consistent basis? A good example of the compound effect would be the following:

The action: I will put aside just €2 every day for a year.
The compound effect: €730 saved at the end of the twelve months.

Maybe your 'action' will be to cut back by one cup of coffee each day and instead replace it with a pint of water. Your actions might be small, but when combined, the results will be significant over a period of time.

The Perfect Day Scenario

When we set goals, they are usually of a materialistic nature: the car, the money, the house… but when you get these materialistic things after a long and hard chase, they're often not what you expected. This disappointment can throw you in a rut, and discourage you from setting more goals. To really establish your ideal goals, just outline what your perfect day would look like.

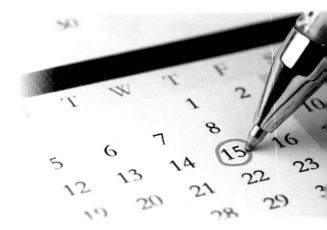

Detail everything that would happen in those 24 hours to make it the most perfect day imaginable. Who would you wake up next to? Who would you spend your time with? Where would you work? What makes the day so perfect? You will probably find that the materialistic things accounted for very little in making this imaginary day perfect. It's just another way of identifying what makes you happy.

Your Support System

One of the most crucial ingredients for success is having the right people around you. A good support system is massively important, so make sure your circle of influence is one that will help keep you motivated. Do what you can to encourage people to join you on your journey, but don't preach to them about healthy foods and workouts. People don't like having someone else's lifestyle forced on them. If they want to make the change, they will do it at their own pace. All you can do is encourage.

If, however, there are people dragging you back or standing in your way, then you need to cut the dead weight. Make the decision to look after yourself first. Sit down with your family and explain the changes you are making to your lifestyle. Don't be afraid to ask them for their support.

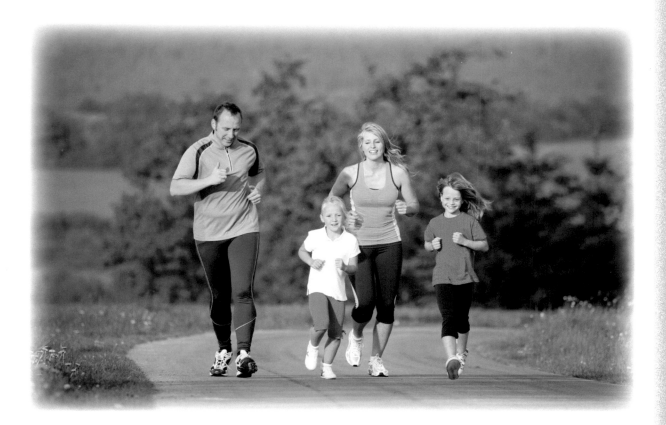

Sometimes one of the biggest 'brakes' can be the person you are living with or hanging around with the most trying to detract you from what you want to do and where you want to be. If your work colleagues are constantly putting biscuits in front of you, then that's a 'brake' and you need to look at how you can change that.

Similarly, if your friends are out drinking, you can go out with them and remain sober, but then you may be making life difficult for yourself by surrounding yourself with temptation. It might be easier to instead seek out people with goals similar to yours. Replace an old activity with a more productive new one. Surround yourself with people who will steer you closer to your goal, not tempt you away from it. If you know what you want, then you will know what actions you should be taking, and what people you should be surrounding yourself with.

Magda and Radek are the perfect example of a good support system. They have completely transformed their lifestyles, and, while it was a huge transition, they supported and encouraged each other throughout. Things like cooking became so much easier because they were doing it together. Their joint goal was their wedding so they were constantly lining each other up for success. Here is their story.

Magda and Radek Mika (Poland)

Our adventure with PDF started in January 2013 and it has turned into the best decision of our lives. It was really hard at the beginning but the most important thing was that we were doing it together, every single day. We supported each other and that give us the power to keeping fighting. After the first month there was no more, "Are we doing next month?", the only question was, "When is the next month starting?"

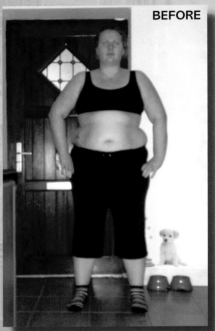

BEFORE

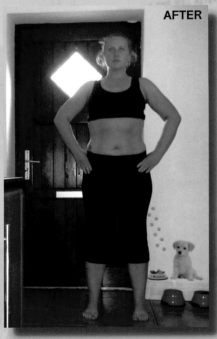

AFTER

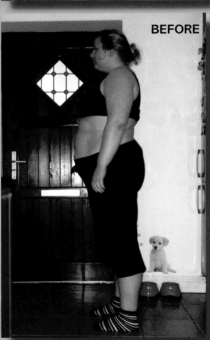

BEFORE

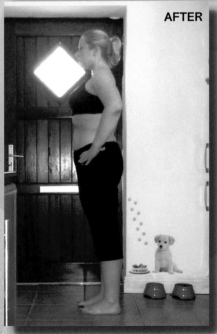

AFTER

Today, we have six months behind us and every pound and inch we lose is just an added benefit. It's no longer diet or exercise, it's our new healthy lifestyle! We have met some amazing people who have become our friends and we get the best support from them and of course from Pat. These changes that we have made in our lives have also brought us even closer in our relationship! We have both fallen in love with fitness, it is now our passion that we share and that has given us a connection like never before... sweat, tears and sacrifice... it's all worth it! Thank you so much Pat for changing our lives into the best lives that we can have!

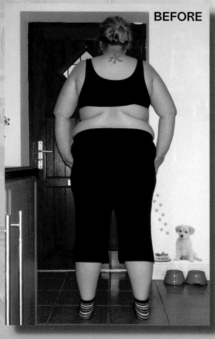
BEFORE

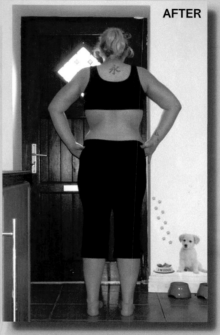
AFTER

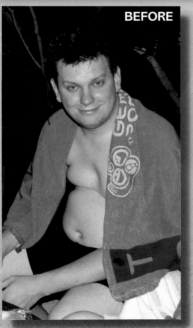
BEFORE

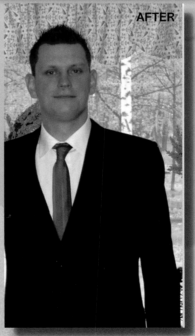
AFTER

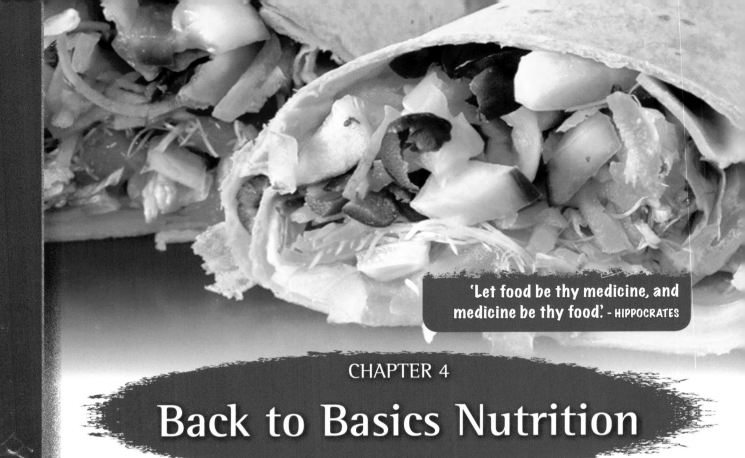

'Let food be thy medicine, and medicine be thy food.' - HIPPOCRATES

CHAPTER 4

Back to Basics Nutrition

I don't believe in calorie counting, or even weighing or measuring foods. Instead I encourage my clients to remove toxic foods such as gluten, dairy, sugar and processed goods from their diets and replace them with real, natural, organic food sources. When it comes to dropping body fat, nutrition is by a clear mile the most important variable. The foods you consume are the building blocks of every piece of you. In the same way that you would not put petrol into a diesel car, we cannot expect our bodies to perform optimally when fuelling them with the wrong food types. First, it's important that we change the way we think about food. Too many of us use food as a comforter or a means of changing our emotions. It is worth asking yourself the next time you want a snack or treat, "Am I actually hungry or am I looking to change the way I feel?"

Instead of thinking of food as a reward, treat or comfort blanket we need to see it for what it really is – fuel for our bodies. This is not to say we shouldn't enjoy food, it is of course one of life's most simple pleasures. But by knowing the 'fuels' which are best for our 'engines' we can eat freely without worrying about calories or weight, comfortable in the knowledge we are allowing ourselves the best chance of looking and feeling our best whilst staying free from illness.

The 'conventional' approach to dropping weight involves cutting back on calories and carbs, weighing and measuring foods and consuming low calorie processed foods and drinks (which contain toxins). This whole approach feeds into the idea that if you burn more calories than you consume you'll drop body fat. But as we've seen, despite the increased availability of low calorie processed foods we are getting fatter and sicker. The problem here is that though you may initially drop weight on a calorie-restricted diet, you are now left with a higher concentration of toxins in a smaller body. To protect itself, the body will store these toxins in fat cells. These fat cells will become stubborn areas which the body doesn't want to let go of and you will end up piling back on additional weight. This is why people get caught in the yo-yo dieting trap. In order to experience lasting results and effective weight control we need to remove these toxins from the body. This is the first step in creating our 'winning environment' for fat loss and health.

In order to experience sustainable weight loss we need to remove toxins from the body.

Every food we consume will either make us healthier or sicker. The right 'fuel' will leave us feeling energised, awake, and ready to take on the day. The wrong 'fuel' (containing toxins) will leave us feeling tired, sluggish, bloated, and lethargic. Our caveman ancestors evolved on a diet mainly made up of meats and seafood, in-season fruits and vegetables, nuts and seeds. This provided them with the energy they needed to hunt and gather all day whilst staying strong, lean and quick. They also lived free from all the diseases that plague modern civilization. We'll look to stick pretty closely to following this 'caveman' style diet during our programme.

That means we'll be looking to eliminate:

- Gluten and legumes

- Sugar

- Dairy

- Alcohol

- Processed foods

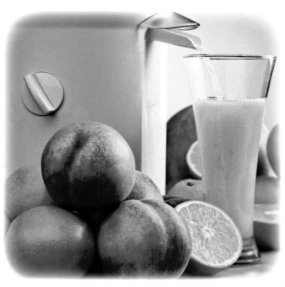

These 'man-made' foods which have come about in the last 10,000 years (the blink of an eye in the greater scheme of things) are the most common allergens which cause all sorts of problems including:

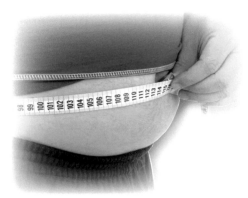

- Abdominal bloating

- Fatigue

- Skin problems

- Low energy levels

- Diarrhoea or constipation

- Mental health problems

- Excessive weight gain

You may look at this list of foods and argue that you consume some or all of the groups listed on a daily basis and don't experience any negative side effects. For me, the only true way of seeing the affect they have on the way you feel and function is to remove them from your diet for 14-21 days before slowly reintroducing them. Sometimes when we have been consistently consuming a certain food (which may be an allergen) for a long period of time we become less aware of how it makes us feel.

It's a bit like walking in to a perfume shop. When you first walk in the smell of perfume is overwhelming, but, the longer you stay, the less noticeable it becomes. Eventually, you no longer notice the smell of perfume at all. Now, if you were to walk out of the shop and back in you would again get the strong smell of perfume. Similarly, sometimes if we are eating a food on an on-going basis we become less and less aware of how our body is reacting to that food. When we remove certain foods and reintroduce them we can quickly highlight the foods that energise us and the foods that leave us feeling sluggish and bloated.

After the 21 days, gluten and dairy can be slowly re-introduced to see how your body handles them. Everybody is different and they might not cause you any problems, but, I'm confident by day 22 most of you will be feeling and functioning so much better without them that you will only want them on occasion as part of a 'cheat meal'.

Let's have a closer look at the foods on our 'banned' list for the duration of the *21 Day Jump Start*.

'The doctor of the future will no longer treat the human frame with drugs, but rather will cure and prevent disease with nutrition.' - THOMAS EDISON

Gluten

In recent years we've been pushed towards increasing our intake of grains and in particular 'healthy' whole grains, the food group most prevalent on the government's recommended food pyramid. Fat was wrongly outlawed as the cause of increased levels of obesity and wholegrain carbohydrate highlighted as the solution. These grains will more often than not contain wheat and wheat will always contain gluten.

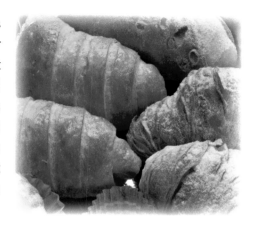

Gluten, a type of 'lectin' is a protein found in wheat, rye, oats and barley. It is most prevalent in wheat, the most popular grain in the Western world. Gluten will be most commonly found in beer, processed or packaged foods, dressings, sauces, soups and fried foods. A significant percentage of the population will experience a gluten intolerance meaning they don't have the enzymes necessary to digest it. I'm sure you've come across a friend of family member who suffers from coeliac disease, an autoimmune disease which has become familiar in recent years. This is gluten intolerance at its most severe. When someone suffering from coeliac disease eats foods containing gluten, damage occurs to the lining of the small intestine. This hinders future absorption of foods and can eventually lead to more serious problems such as malnutrition. (It's worth noting that plenty of us actually suffer from symptoms of coeliac disease or gluten intolerance without knowing it.) Less severe cases of gluten intolerance may present symptoms such as abdominal bloating, digestive problems, diarrhoea, constipation, gas or low energy levels.

As we have become more health conscious in recent years, food marketers have looked to capitalise with 'gluten-free' alternatives. Much like the 'low fat, low calorie' foods which have become popular in recent years it must be noted that 'gluten-free' and 'healthy' do not necessarily go hand in hand. These foods are often heavily processed and contain blood-sugar-elevating alternatives to gluten.

Like wheat, legumes and beans contain phytates which are indigestible agents. These phytates inhibit the absorption of zinc, magnesium, calcium and iron. This means you might be making a conscious effort to get all of your crucial minerals in food or supplement form but you are actually preventing yourself from absorbing them.

During our programme we'll be removing gluten in order to allow ourselves a better understanding of how our bodies function in its absence. We'll also remove beans and legumes for the 3 weeks. I've had many clients experience increased energy levels and improved digestion in a matter of weeks by simply omitting foods containing gluten from their meals. Clients suffering from irritable bowel syndrome (IBS) have commonly reported massive improvements.

Sugar

Sugar is a highly addictive drug.

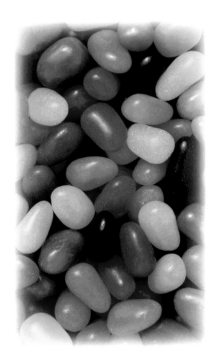

Sugar acts in much the same way as heroin, releasing increased amounts of dopamine, the neurotransmitter responsible for energy, memory and focus. Comparing sugar to heroin might sound crazy but it can't be denied that the majority of the population suffer from a sugar addiction, an addiction that's making us fat and sick. This isn't surprising when you consider the fact that most of us have been consuming it in large quantities from a very young age. With the exception of honey, little refined sugar was available up until around 400 years ago but today sugar makes up a large percentage of our daily food intake.

When we consume sugar (glucose), the liver will store this glucose as glycogen for energy at a later time. The liver can only store around 100g of glucose before it has to be stored elsewhere. When we have excess glycogen, it is returned to the blood stream and stored as body fat.

As well as the likelihood of storing excess body fat from excess sugar intake, a small percentage of the population will have an hereditary fructose intolerance. This intolerance can also develop as a result of over-consumption of processed sugars, sweeteners and fruit.

It's worth noting that a 'natural' sugar is still a sugar, and your body handles it the same way.

For the next 21 days, I'd like you to cut out all sugar including:

- High glycemic fruits
- Honey
- Syrups
- High fructose corn syrup
- Table sugar
- Sucrose
- Fizzy drinks
- Sports drinks
- Powdered sugar
- Agave nectar

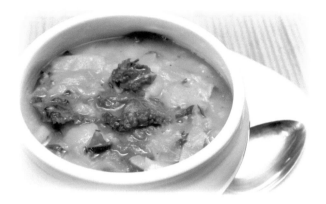

Dairy

Much like wholegrains, dairy, particularly milk, has always been considered a staple of a healthy diet. Since childhood we've been encouraged to drink milk to be healthy and strong. It may, however, be another problematic food type for many of us.

Milk products contain lactose, a natural sugar which is digested by the enzyme 'lactase'. Essential enzymes are removed in the process of pasteurisation and homogenisation in order to prolong shelf life. In the process of homogenisation the milk or milk product is heated to remove all harmful bacteria. Unfortunately, at the same time, key minerals, amino acids and enzymes are also removed. Many of us are deficient in lactase, making the digestion of foods containing lactose impossible. Common symptoms of a lactose intolerance include acne, eczema, abdominal cramping, bloating, headaches, joint pains, congestion and nausea. Again, by removing dairy products from our diet for the 21 days and then slowly reintroducing them we will have a much better idea of how our bodies react to lactose and milk products. An interesting fact for you – humans are the only mammal who drink the milk of another mammal.

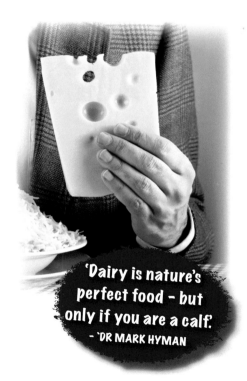

'Dairy is nature's perfect food – but only if you are a calf.'
- DR MARK HYMAN

Those who are lactose intolerant will sometimes do okay with raw, unsweetened, and unpasteurised dairy. Butter, full cream, cottage cheese, full fat Greek-style yogurt, and, raw whole milk, can be added to your meals, but at no point, should they become a centrepiece within your diet.

Some of you are probably worried that your bones will fall apart when you remove dairy from the diet! We've been taught since school that the calcium found in milk is responsible for strong, healthy bones. It's interesting to note that the countries with the lowest rates of dairy and calcium consumption also share the lowest rates of osteoporosis.

Full fat Greek-style yogurt will be okay for most, even those who struggle to digest dairy. This is due to the fact it's yeast culture eats the lactose in the milk. Avoid 'low-fat' or flavoured alternatives and opt only for full fat organic natural yogurt.

Alcohol

We all enjoy a drink (or ten) after a tough week at the office! Unfortunately, for those of us why enjoy a 'tipple', alcohol has no positive bearing on our health or weight loss efforts. Even a beverage branded as

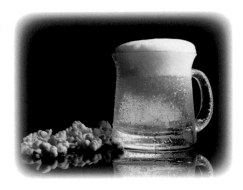

'Here's to alcohol; the cause of, and solution to, all of life's problems.'
– HOMER SIMPSON

gluten free or 'low' in calories contains alcohol, so whichever way you choose to look at it you are still ingesting a toxin which provides nothing but empty calories. It's loaded with sugar and places extra stress on the kidneys, liver and adrenal glands. Regular alcohol consumption can also result in damage to the stomach wall and lining, resulting in leaky gut syndrome. Claims that some drinks, like red wine, having amazing health benefits, are little more than clever marketing by drinks companies. Sorry to be the bearer of bad news!

I'm not saying I expect you to never drink again (I wouldn't do that to you... or me!), but it's important that instead of fooling ourselves, we know the true effect alcohol has on our weight loss and improved health efforts. This again puts us in a position of power where we can make smarter decisions and not be left wondering why we aren't getting the desired results from our training and nutrition programme.

We talked earlier about hormonal balance being the key to improved health and all the benefits that come with it and we'll talk later about the role sleep plays in getting your hormones in balance for optimal health. Alcohol wreaks havoc on both our sleep patterns and our hormones. It also places additional stress on the liver, our body's detoxifier. One of the liver's prime responsibilities is metabolising fat. If we are drinking alcohol, it takes effort and energy to remove it from your system, leaving you less energy for fat metabolising, muscle recovery and other essential processes that promote optimal health.

Alcohol also affects our natural sleep rhythm and the growth hormone production that comes with it. Growth hormone is responsible for muscle growth, fat loss and general wellbeing. On top of all this, alcohol impairs our decisions and leaves us craving junk food. And you don't need me to tell you that the takeaway at 3am isn't going to move us toward our body transformation goals!

For 21 days we'll cut out all alcohol, no excuses! This is the one people usually fight me on, but you need to commit 100% to the programme as laid out. If you decide to pick and choose which parts you intend to follow, then it's no longer my programme, it's yours, and it is probably not going to work half as well!

Processed Foods

As mentioned earlier, the way we eat has changed more in the last 50 years than it did in the previous 10,000. Food companies are out to make as much money as possible with no regard for public health. Processed foods are the greatest example of this.

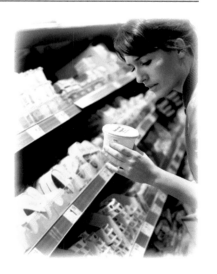

The majority of us will come home from the supermarket each week with grocery bags largely filled with packaged foods which have been heavily processed to prolong their shelf life. These foods are loaded with additives, preservatives and pesticides which are completely foreign to the human body. These same foods contain known carcinogens, so why do we continue to eat them?

Processed foods are very addictive. They over-stimulate our production of dopamine, the pleasure neurotransmitter leaving us wanting more. Also, since they contain so many 'ingredients' that are foreign to the body, we derive little if any nutritional value from them and are left hungry not long after eating.

We are among the first generations to take in this abundance of chemicals and I believe the massive increase in disease in recent years is testament to the fact these processed foods are playing a part in killing us off.

Pat's Comprehensive Guide to Reading Food Labels

If it has a food label, you probably shouldn't be eating it! If the label contains ingredients that are unrecognisable or illegible to you, you definitely shouldn't be eating it!

Insulin – The Master Hormone

Time for a little lesson in endocrinology. I'll keep it very straightforward and hopefully leave you with a better understanding of how we get fat and sick from consuming too much carbohydrate (sugar).

We spoke a little about sugar, it's addictive properties and the resulting fat gain that comes from excessive consumption of sugar from a variety of sources. We also briefly touched on the importance of hormonal balance in our pursuit of weight loss and overall health. The two main hormones in relation to storage and release of energy in the body are insulin and glucagon. You may have heard of insulin, possibly in relation to diabetes. When we eat, insulin helps us store food to be used as energy at a later date. This is first stored in the liver and once the liver reaches its storage capacity is kept as body fat throughout

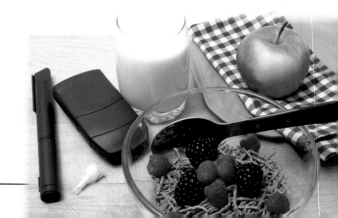

the body. Glucagon does the opposite to insulin, allowing us to use our stored energy at a later time after we have eaten.

Now, the problem is that most of us are in an insulin dominant state the majority of the time. This triggers some detrimental processes in the body. Firstly, the insulin turns our metabolism to storage mode and causes us to store more and more food energy as fat. This insulin also switches on our cholesterol synthesis system causing us to produce more cholesterol. Most of the cholesterol in our bodies we produce ourselves, only around 20-30% comes from dietary cholesterol. We'll talk more about cholesterol later and look at how we can lower it easily without medication through dietary recommendations which you probably wouldn't expect.

Our goal with the *21 Day Jump Start* is to get our hormonal balance back in check and switch our body from a fat storing machine to a fat releasing machine.

Another 'Low Carb' Diet?

Many of you may look at the programme and see it as another 'low carb' diet at first. Low carb diets get a bit of a bit of a bad rap and sometimes justifiably so. Cutting back on carbohydrate makes dropping weight easy in the short term. You'll probably drop some body fat and undoubtedly some retained water but often low carb dieters will find themselves piling weight back on or plateauing before reaching their desired weight and shape.

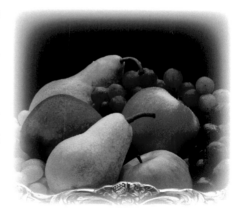

The problem with many low carb diets is that they focus only on weight loss and not on pursuing health. Remember, weight loss is simply a side effect of good health, so we always focus on health first. They often contain an abundance of fats and not enough protein. Low carb diets also drastically drop calories and don't place enough emphasis on the quality of the proteins and fats being taken in. This leaves the dieter feeling tired, run-down and miserable. What good is it being lean if you feel like crap?

It's worth noting that 'low-carb' is relative to the individual, their current condition and their activity levels. Again, let's go back to the analogy of your body being an engine and this time carbohydrate being its fuel. On a short journey you will need only a small amount of fuel, but for a long trip you will need a full tank. In much the same way, when your activity levels are relatively low you won't need as much carbohydrate whereas when you are setting out to do an endurance race or marathon you may benefit from taking in a lot more carbohydrate.

For most of us, our lifestyles are much more sedentary than say the lifestyles of our grandparents during their earlier years. Less active lifestyles should call for less 'fuel' but as we all know this isn't the case. Carbohydrates, regardless of their source, convert to sugar and we are taking in more sugar than ever before.

For the course of the *21 Day Jump Start* we will be cutting out refined sugar, processed foods and excess carbohydrate. Instead we will focus on taking in good sources of proteins, fats, low glycemic fruits and vegetables with the intention of bringing your body back to a place where it has natural energy that can support your activity levels whilst burning excess body fat.

So What Can I Eat?

I know what you're thinking! I've asked you to cut out gluten, dairy, alcohol, sugar and processed foods for the next 21 days and you probably feel like I've left you with nothing but rabbit food to eat. Don't worry, I wouldn't do that to you! It may take you a few days to get into the swing of things with the new shopping list and guidelines but I'm confident you'll come to love this new way of eating and the way it makes you feel. 21 days has been outlined as the amount of time it takes to form a new habit and I'm confident if you stick to the foods on the shopping list you'll carry forward these healthy habits through day 22 and beyond.

As I mentioned in the introduction, this is about creating a lifestyle that is enjoyable and sustainable. There won't be any calorie counting, measuring or weighing foods. We're just going to take a straightforward approach to detoxing the body, loading up on great nutrients and bringing the body's natural hormonal balance back to where it should be. When we do this (and it's not difficult to do) we almost instantly see improvements in energy levels, sleep, appearance and wellbeing. We also experience effortless weight loss.

Structuring your meals couldn't be easier. Portion control isn't a concern (within reason) and you'll never be left hungry!

Meals will be made up of a protein source, a large serving of greens and a source of healthy fats. On top of this there will be room for snacks where desired. Before going through exactly how to put your meals together let's briefly look at what we are looking to include in each meal and why they're needed.

Examples of healthy fats: Avocados, yolk of an egg, nuts, seeds, goats cheese, feta cheese, coconut oils, olive oils.

Protein

Proteins are the building blocks of the human body, which means that in order to have a strong and healthy body, muscles, blood, teeth and skin, adequate protein intake from good quality sources is essential. In recent years. supplement companies marketing to bodybuilders and athletes have stressed the importance of protein intake for optimal health, growth and recovery. To think that these protein requirements are only needed for elite athletes and bodybuilders would be a mistake. Protein is just as important for the 'average Joe or Jane'. Your body completely rebuilds itself every year. The skin, liver, stomach lining, brain, blood and body. With proteins being the building blocks for this constant growth and repair of the human body the expression 'you are what you eat' could not be a truer statement. The starting point for every meal during your programme is a high quality protein source.

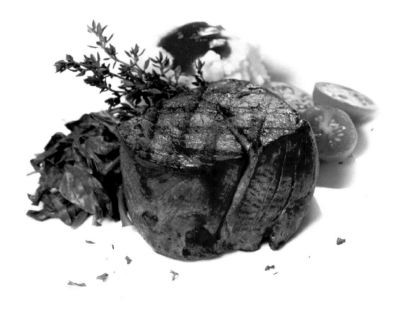

Meat/Poultry	Fish/Seafood	Miscellaneous

• Beef
• Buffalo
• Elk
• Heart
• Kidney
• Lamb
• Liver (Beef)
• Rabbit
• Venison
• Chicken (Dark Meat)
  Chicken (White Meat)
• Hen
• Duck
• Goose
• Pheasant
• Quail
• Turkey (Dark Meat)
  Turkey (White Meat)
	• Salmon
	• Sardines
	• Anchovy
	• Bass (Freshwater)
	  Sea bass
	• Cod
	• Crayfish
	• Haddock
	• Halibut
	• Herring
	• Oysters
	• Shrimp/Prawns
	• Scallops
	• Snapper
	• Trout
	• Clams
	• Crab
	• Lobster
	• Mackerel
	• Mussels
	• Squid
	• Swordfish
	• Tuna (fresh)
		• Eggs (Chicken)
		• Eggs (Duck)
		• Whey Protein Powder
		• Casein Protein Powder
		• Rice/Pea/Hemp Protein
		  Powder
		• Cottage Cheese

Fats

Fats have been villified over the years and wrongly labelled as the cause of obesity and health problems related to being overweight. They have also been held responsible for the prominence of high cholesterol and high blood pressure in today's population. In reality, it's sugar that is the problem, and always has been. Fat doesn't make you fat, sugar does! Consuming the right types of fats can actually have a tremendous impact on your health and your weight loss efforts. Healthy fats are essential for healthy hormones. They will also ramp up your metabolism and keep you full for longer.

A common mistake among dieters is dropping their calories dramatically by cutting out carbohydrates. Yet they don't replace these lost calories with an energy source. It is essential that we add healthy fats to suppress appetite and provide a source of energy. If we cut out carbohydrate and sugar without adding in some additional healthy fats our bodies go into 'survival mode' and hold onto the fat we've got, out of fear that there is very little food coming in! You'll also feel run down, sluggish and completely drained of energy. Not what you want!

We've already spoken about the rise in availability of 'low fat' foods. We've also seen a tremendous rise in larger waistlines across the population. There is no coincidence here. When you remove the fat from a food you will tend to remove a lot of the taste. In order to replace this taste, sugar, additives and preservatives are added to these 'low fat foods'. Ironically, it's the sugar and processed additions that make these 'low fat' foods so fattening.

Now this is not to say all fats are good. Trans fats, hydrogenated fats and some saturated fats are bad news.

Trans fats or hydrogenated fats are processed fats which are cheap and have a prolonged shelf-life, making them very popular. They are found in many foods including pizzas, pastries, pies, crackers, salad dressings and cookies. They will also more often than not be found in fried foods. These, along with cheap cooking oils, are obviously the fats we are looking to avoid.

Instead, during our programme and beyond, I'd like you to focus on 'good fats' found in foods such as avocados, nuts, seeds, nut butters, and oily fish. These fats help to lower bad cholesterol and boost metabolism. They also help to lower bad cholesterol (low-density lipoprotein).

Nuts/Seeds/Nut Butters	Fish/Seafood	Oils/Miscellaneous
• Raw and unsalted, no peanuts! • Almonds • Brazil nuts • Cashews • Chestnuts • Macadamias • Pecans • Pine nuts • Pistachios • Walnuts • Pumpkin seeds • Sesame seeds • Flax seeds • Chia seeds • Almond nut butter • Cashew nut butter • Hazelnut Butter	• Herring • Mackerel • Salmon • Sardines • Swordfish • Trout • Tuna steaks	• Coconut oil • Evening primrose oil • Fish oil • Flax seed oil • Hemp oil • Walnut oil • Avocado oil • Extra Virgin Olive oil • Omega 3 enriched eggs • Grass-fed meats

People have become obsessed with eating certain foods at certain times of the day. For instance, they associate cereals with breakfast. On that note, if you are starting each day with a bowl of cereal, you are setting yourself up for weight gain because you are effectively telling your body to store fat for the day. Believe it or not, stir fried fish cooked in coconut oil, or steak with nuts, and a portion of mixed vegetables would be the best breakfast you could possibly have. It's a psychological adjustment. People need to stop thinking of fish and steak as being dinner foods only.

Supplements

The diet and fitness industry is a massive business that grosses billions every year. The supplement companies are among the biggest earners in the industry, supplying thousands of formulas for potions, pills and powders with promises of life-changing results. In reality, much of the stock on shelves is little more than cleverly marketed, overpriced junk. Add to that the fact that many of the formulas previously available have been discontinued due to health risks and you may re-think forking out your hard-earned cash for little more than empty promises and potential health risks.

With that being said, there are some quality supplements available on the market which I would highly recommend to you. Do remember that diet always comes number one. You can't out-supplement or out-train a bad diet!

Coconut Oil

To me, this isn't really a supplement. In fact, it should be a part of everyone's regular shopping list but I thought I'd stick it in here anyway. I'm delighted to see coconut oil being made more readily available in supermarkets as well as specialist health stores. It's an amazing resource with countless health benefits!

What does it do?
There are so many health benefits associated with the use of coconut oil! One of the beauties of using coconut oil is that it holds a very high smoking point meaning it can be used for cooking at high temperatures. This is of particular importance when cooking on the pan. Other oils including olive oil oxidise at high temperatures creating free radicals which we don't want. The

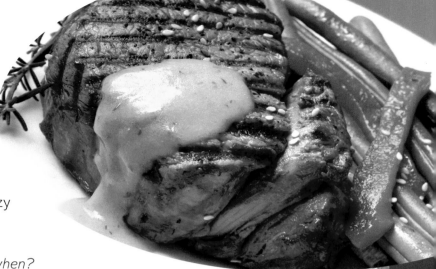

good fats in coconut oil also make it great for preventing sugar cravings and keeping you fuller for longer. Add to this the fact that coconut oil improves digestion, skin, hair, nails and ramps up your metabolism and you'd be crazy not to start using it!

How much should I take and when?
I would encourage you to use a generous amount of coconut oil for all of your cooking. You can also add a tablespoon to your coffee or green tea for a natural boost and serving of good fats. 1-3 tablespoons per day (including that used whilst cooking) is recommended.

Omega 3 Fish Oil
What does it do?
A key factor in attaining and maintaining good health is the balance of our intake of Omega 3 and Omega 6 fatty acids. While our caveman ancestors would have taken in a ratio of omega-6 to omega-3 close to 1:1 we are now taking in anywhere from 15:1 to 20:1.

Omega 6's are found in a lot of cheap oils and processed foods which have become a staple of many diets. Supplementing with Omega 3 fish oil is a convenient way of helping bring the balance back to where it should be.

Omega 3's, EPA and DHA improve brain function and help decrease inflammation.

How much should I take and when?
Dosages will vary dependent on the concentration and brand of oil you buy. The main thing you should be looking for when purchasing a fish oil, whether it's in liquid or capsule form, is the EPA and DHA content. These are the key ingredients. Your total intake of combined EPA and DHA for the day should be in around 3g minimum. An oil or capsules containing less than 500mg combined EPA and DHA per serving is low quality and should be avoided.

Wheatgrass

What does it do?

You probably remember learning about the pH scale in school? One end of the spectrum is extremely acidic, the other end extremely alkaline. Stress, poor diet, alcohol and other external toxins leave our bodies in a very acidic state where we cannot experience optimal health or weight loss. Unfortunately, the majority of the foods we are buying are on the acidic side of the scale. When your body's pH level is balanced, you will notice improved energy levels, sleep and overall wellbeing as well as the loss of any unwanted excess body fat. Dark, leafy green vegetables are among the most alkaline foods on the planet and wheatgrass provides this same alkaline effect in a much more concentrated dosage.

How much should I take and when?

I recommend a teaspoon of wheatgrass in water once to twice daily to help alkalise the body. If you are currently in a very acidic state you may find the wheatgrass tough to stomach. This gets better as your body becomes more alkaline (and as I always tell my clients who complain about the taste, I'm sure you've drank a lot worse on a night out on the town)!

Glutamine

What does it do?

Glutamine is the most abundant amino acid in the human body (amino acids being the building blocks of protein). In the bodybuilding and fitness community it's been marketed and used as a supplement for muscle recovery after tough workouts but add to that the benefits of improved gut health and immunity and you'll see why I'm a big believer in glutamine.

How much should I take and when?

Glutamine is found in both powder and tablet form, but I want you to get the one in powder form. Take a teaspoon first thing in the morning, and another last thing at night.

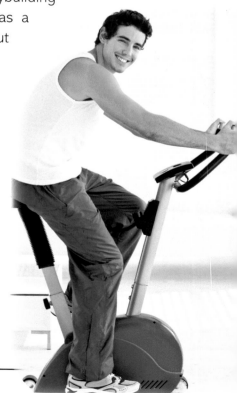

Mark Quinn (Athlone, Co Westmeath)

Pat helped me change my way of thinking towards training and diet. I had been training for years for events like triathlons and half marathons, while also hitting the gym two or three times a week, but yet, I wasn't getting the results I expected. I was under the impression that I could eat anything I wanted as I was running up to 40km per week. I was wrong!

I noticed Pat's programme one evening on Facebook and thought I'd give it a go. It turned out to be the best money I've ever spent. From the programme I learned all about eating clean and that having a good diet is way more important than actually working out, I know now that it's probably 75% diet and 25% working out. I also learned about High Intensity Interval Training, which meant I would work harder for a shorter period of time rather than heading off on a long steady run. This saved me time in the evenings to sit back and relax and also I couldn't believe the results. Thanks again Pat.

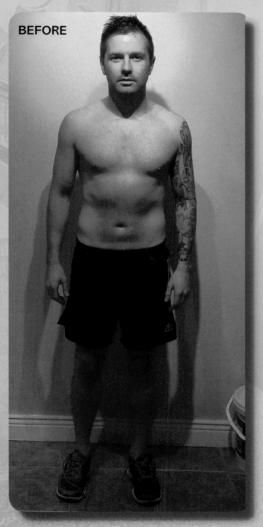
BEFORE

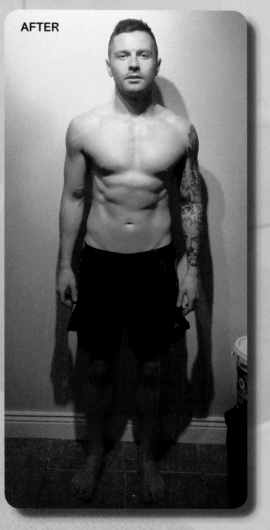
AFTER

WATER TIME

2 glasses of water in the morning will help rev up your metabolism for the day.

1 glass of water half an hour before a meal will help digestion.

1 glass of water before taking a bath will helps lower blood pressure

1 glass of water before bed will also help prevent night time leg cramps.

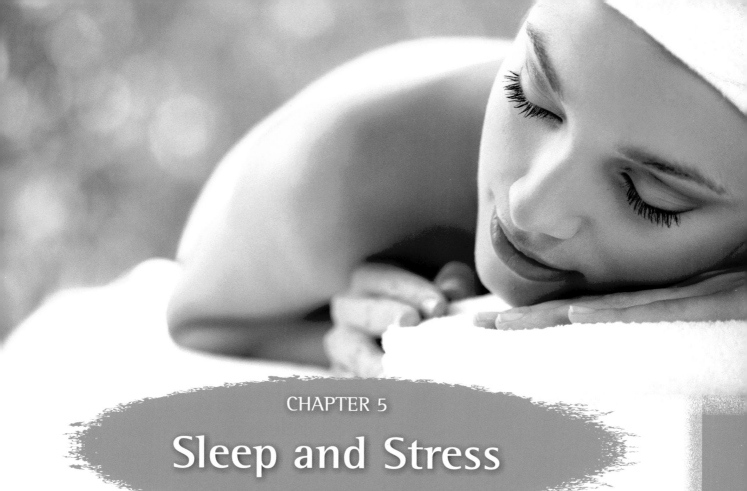

CHAPTER 5

Sleep and Stress

Stress has become one of the biggest killers of our generation. Again, it comes back to cave man ancestors. Their way of living is completely foreign to us. They had situations of acute stress but these were always over very quickly. When a cave man was attacked by a wild animal, he had that fight or flight response. It was a situation of great stress but it would pass within a couple of minutes.

Our bodies cannot tell the difference between the various types of stressors. The stress we experience when we are stuck in traffic has the same affect on our bodies as it did on that of the caveman when he was being attacked by a wild animal. In today's world however, the stress is constant. It doesn't pass. Our alarm clock going off in the morning is a stressor, fighting with a family member is a stressor, your boss being a bully is a stressor. The stress hormone is cortisol. Ideally your cortisol levels should be higher in the morning. This is what gets you up and energised. Cortisol levels usually peak at around 3pm, and then, as the day goes on, they begin to get lower, which is when you relax and unwind. People are so stressed, however, that their cortisol levels are through the roof. It doesn't help that they are adding

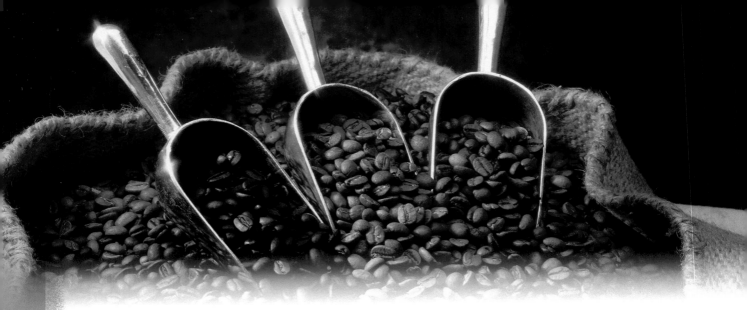

stimulants like coffee and sugar, which raise cortisol levels. It's a vicious circle where your cortisol levels are not winding down like they should and you end up being tired but wired! You feel shattered at the end of the day and you want to sleep but you can't because you are highly caffeinated. When you get up the following morning, you are wrecked and this is because your cortisol levels are not high when they should be. You find it hard to get going in the mornings, so you load up on coffee which again brings your cortisol levels out of balance. Ideally, you should be getting up when the sun is rising, and going to bed when the sun is setting.

During the summer, our ancestors would have eaten a lot of fruit in order to bulk up in preparation for the winter. They would also have experienced a lot of carbohydrate cravings during these long summer days. A consequence of modern day artificial lighting, however, is that our bodies think it's summer, and so this is why we get carb cravings in the evening and late at night.

The Sleep Tight Routine

Aim to rise between 6am and 9am. During the day, you can bring your cortisol levels down naturally by avoiding caffeine after 2pm, and dimming down the lights in the house a few hours before going to bed. Alcohol and nicotine will also affect your sleep cycle so try to cut down on them as much as possible. If you need help relaxing at night, try drinking some Tulsi Tea. Magnesium, likewise, is a good supplement that will help you unwind. Try to turn off the computer and the TV at least an hour before bed. Maybe replace these activities with some light and easy reading. Darken the room as much as possible. Any brightness in the room will make your body think it's still day time and it won't want to shut off. Try to get to bed by 10.30pm/11pm.

Cortisol can lead to an increased storage of fat around the stomach area. When people can't seem to drop the fat from their belly or love handles, the problem is often related to sleep and stress problems. You might be getting the food and fitness aspects right, but if your sleep routine isn't right, then you won't see results in the stomach area.

On that note, forget the diet pills. They are generally caffeine-based stimulants, so while they might bump up your metabolism and heart rate, they will also bump up your cortisol levels which will make if difficult to get a good sleep.

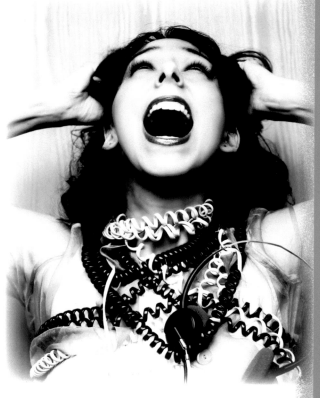

Digital Detox

A major contributing factor to our stress levels is how accessible we have become. This makes it very hard to switch off. We can be contacted via text, phone calls, Viber, Facebook, Twitter, and email. Our phones have become a 24 hour access point. It used to be the case that when we left the office, we could forget about work until the following morning, but now, there seems to be no switch off. For seven days, try and limit your use of social media and email to fifteen minutes in the morning and fifteen minutes in the evening. Disconnect from the online world. People think they can't live without checking their Facebook pages, but we all survived pretty well for years before it came along, so there is no reason why we can't cut down on it now! It will be difficult at first but you should find it a good de-stressor.

Mairead Vesey (Longford/Roscommon)

I first became aware of Pat Divilly Fitness through Facebook in February 2013, when details of the Project Alpha programme came up on my newsfeed. I 'Liked' his page and became intrigued by this project. I am 34 years old and had been 'thin' up to the birth of my first daughter who is now 8 years old. I have since had two more children, and all three by C section, so needless to say, my stomach muscles were very weak. Since the birth of my son last year, I just thought, that's it, my body would always look like it's gone through the mill and I would never get my tummy area to look normal again. I hated my body.

I really had an urge to get fit in the spring time, and after watching Pat explain his programme on YouTube, I decided to try it. I signed up and enthusiastically got all the supplements and foods on the list, all ready to start on March 4th 2013. The first few days were tough as I went through the detox process, but I was determined to see it through. After a few days with the detox symptoms such as headaches and low energy, I became stronger and was buzzing about with huge energy. I enjoyed the food aspect, loved trying out the various workouts, and I soon started seeing results. In April, when I had my first night out with my family in Sligo, everyone commented on how well I was looking! They noticed my weight loss, and even how clear my skin was. I was delighted, so I vowed to continue with this new lifestyle. In my 16th week, I had lost a total of 23 inches all over and 22 pounds. My mindset regarding food has changed. If I am eating out, I tend to look for the healthy option automatically. I make time to do the workouts; not always an easy task when you have three kids and a full time job, but, with each workout, I seem to get stronger. I have also learned to ignore the weighing scales. These were once a big thing for me, but, I see now its about how the plan shrinks the body rather then how much weight you lose.

I wish to thank Pat Divilly for his help and support so far. I have made huge strides with regard to regaining my confidence and my wedding day figure, something I thought would be impossible! Strangers at work have gone from asking me, 'When are you due?' (when I wasn't even pregnant!), to saying things like, 'You would never guess you've had three children!'

It's the biggest compliment, and Pat has helped me achieve it. I also loved that his private groups on Facebook allowed clients a facility through which to share their experiences and problems with fellow members who were also going through the process. It was a wonderful support system, and I have made some fantastic new friends through it. It's a very different programme to those on the market at present but it certainly works. For his young age, Pat certainly has his head in the right place. He is working so hard to help me and so many others achieve what I personally thought was impossible. From the bottom of my heart, thank you Pat.

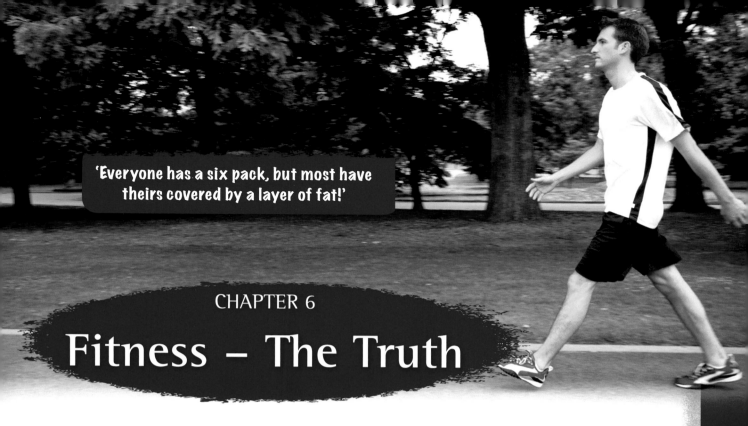

'Everyone has a six pack, but most have theirs covered by a layer of fat!'

CHAPTER 6

Fitness – The Truth

The fitness business is a money-making industry, and it centres around fads and general bullshit. The reality is that nothing has changed over the years in terms of nutrition and fitness. The principles of success still remain the very same. Good marketing, however, makes things seem more complex so as to elicit a need to spend more money on equipment, fads and programmes.

If you want guaranteed success, then forget the fads and return to basics.

The Way to Burn Fat Faster

Strength training is a far better option than cardio when it comes to dropping fat. You will burn so much more this way.

People often spend a long time on the treadmill or the cross trainer doing a massive amount of cardio training. I am more in favour of the high intensity training. People sometimes brag about being able to do two or three hours on the treadmill, but if you can last that long, then you are not pushing yourself hard enough. The key to burning fat is intensity. It's not about the length of time you are running, it's about the intensity. You can go low intensity for days but its high intensity that will give you the desirable results. Look at your typical marathon runner. They can run for a long period of time, but

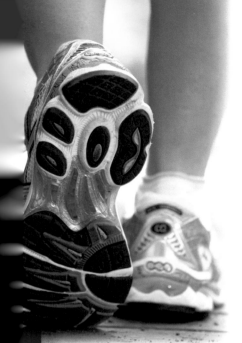

they mostly look frail, almost like they would break in two. Sprinters, on the other hand, can do high intensity sprints over very short periods of time, and they look strong and lean. Sprinters look a lot healthier than most marathon runners and endurance athletes.

Your body adapts to the stress you put on it, so if you train your body to run for two hours each day then it will soon adapt to that and you won't see the changes you want.

High intensity is relative to the individual. On a scale of one to ten, aim to have your high intensity sprints at an eight, your rest period (e.g. jogging) at a level of four. By alternating between periods of high intensity and rest, you are elevating your heart rate to a point where you are still burning calories even after you stop training. It's all because your heart rate has increased. This process is called EPOC, although its better known as after-burn. If you do high intensity training for 45 minutes, you will burn fat for that 45 minutes, but you will also continue burning fat for hours afterwards, even when you are sitting watching television. With low intensity training, you are burning a small amount when you train, but you burn nothing when you stop.

If you trained really intensely, your body could very possibly continue burning fat for twelve hours after that training session. Try to train your whole body, not just specific muscles. Some people have a weak back because they do so much stomach work. Work with full body movements. If you are working bigger muscle groups, you are burning more calories.

You are always going to have an element of soreness when you start training. No amount of warming up will prevent this. Stretching out will help, as will Epsom salt baths, but your body will still feel a little sore after the first day or two.

Don't get distracted by different fads, if you want to run a 10k race, then train like a 10k runner. You don't need to be doing obstacle courses and other crazy fads or diets. If you get caught up in the complexity of training, you will quickly lose interest. Everything in your plan should be there for a reason. Every step of your plan should have a purpose. If every exercise and every rest period has its own purpose then it makes for a very efficient plan. There is too much circus training going on at the moment. People are getting

caught up in crazy fads that either sell because they have a shock factor, or else they are being endorsed by celebrities. Get back to basics, however, and you will get results.

Flexibility and Mobility

Mobility and flexibility are two ignored issues. You lose the flexibility and mobility you had as kid, and it steadily gets worse as you age. People blame old age, but it's actually a result of the way they have been living. There are plenty of elderly people doing yoga and going swimming and they move perfectly well! They have trained their bodies to think that these activities are standard routine. If you sit down all the time, you are conditioning your body to do only that. Again, your body will adapt to whatever stress you put upon it.

You live in a convenience culture. You sit at the breakfast table in the morning, you sit into the car to go to work, you sit at the office desk, you sit down for lunch, you sit into the car to drive home, you sit down for dinner, you then most likely sit down for the evening watching soaps. When people do go to the gym, they tend to sit down on machines, but this is the last thing they should be doing! One of the new silent killers is the amount of time people are sitting down each day. It leads to lower back and hip problems. Personally, I like to get my clients moving in the way they should be moving. If you watch a toddler, they can move they way we should be moving. They have good mobility and flexibility, they can squat with perfect balance because they learn from the ground up. Modern day living conditions us to almost be immobile and de-conditioned. Again, your body adapts to whatever stress you put on it. If you are teaching your body to sit down all the time, then its going to adapt! Your posture will suffer as will your back. Your hips will tighten. If you spend most of your day seated, then stay away from seated equipment in the gym otherwise you are only making your weak points weaker. People also tend to train in front of a mirror, and, consequently they only train the front of the body. Its crucial that you train your back muscles as well! Basic human functions are things like squatting, lunging, walking, twisting, turning, these actions mirror real life. People are suffering from different injuries and ailments like back pain because they are not strong enough in proper plains of motion. Rely less on the equipment and concentrate more on handling your own body weight. For instance, you are likely to squat down to pick something off the floor, so squatting is one exercise that mimics a real life motion.

Improving your flexibility

When you are watching TV, make it a habit to get down and do a few stretches every time an ad break comes on.

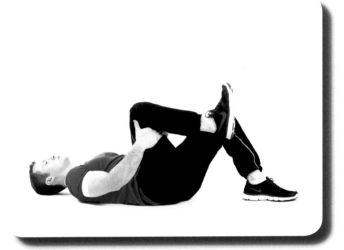

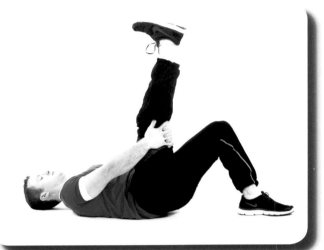

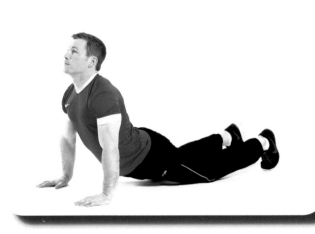

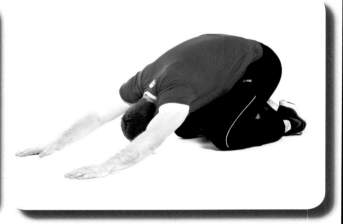

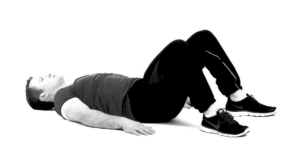

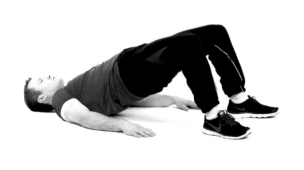

Strength is more important than fitness

Once you get strong, fitness will follow. You lose muscle as you get older, and this is why strength training is important. It will also make a huge difference between a minor and major injury if in the event you should take a fall.

The Elements of a Good Training Programme

- Flexibility and mobility

- Strength training

- Core conditioning

- Cardiovascular training (to help build up pace)

The Six Pack Myth

Many assume that sit-up exercises are the best way to uncover this six-pack. They're not! You can do sit-ups for hours each day, but they will have no benefit if your diet isn't right. I, personally, am not a fan of sit-up exercises because they just mimic being seated, which is something I try to move people away from. If you want to tone the stomach area, then plank exercises are far more effective than sit-ups.

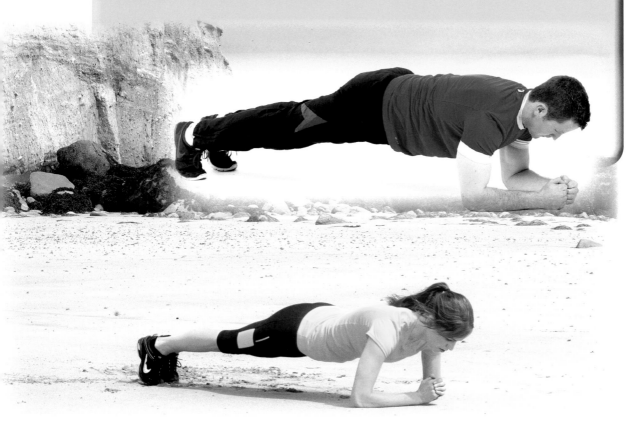

Body transformations don't happen overnight. Attaining your absolutely ideal physique can take many weeks, months, and sometimes years. The best diet or training plan in the world cannot suddenly counteract years of neglect on your body. You don't lose weight over the course of a handful of days, much like you didn't gain weight over a handful of days. Weight loss, just like weight gain, is the accumulation of years of habits, be they good or bad. Consistency, however, is king when it comes to making changes to your body. It may take you longer than others, you may hit plateaus or feel you aren't progressing at the rate you'd like to, but keep plugging away by making good food choices and being physically active. Take care of your body, and, over time you will see amazing changes.

CLIENT TESTIMONIAL

Adrian Hanley (Galway)

I started off at 19st 1lb last October [2012]. I got my hands on Pat's 14 Day Detox, which he had kindly given away for free through Facebook, and, through that, I learned a huge amount about my body and what I should or should not be eating. I found it tough, but, as the saying goes, Rome wasn't built in a day. It takes a lot of motivation and self confidence to do Pat's programme. He gives you the tools, but you have to work at it. A lot of people promise this, that, and the other, but I feel Pat's approach is fantastic. If you follow it and trust the process you will achieve what you want. I started the classes, as I wanted something different and structured during the week. The classes are just the best. Never in my life did I think I would be as fit as I am at this moment in time. I owe it all to the classes. Pat is a superb mentor not just to myself but to everyone in the class. He always answers my questions, and I always have many, be it about technique, diet, or training. I'm now doing 28KG kettle bell swings, 10K runs and many other exercises I never thought I would be able to do.

I don't want to sound corny or cheesy but being part of PDF has changed my life. I'm fitter, healthier, relaxed, and far more confident since I started it all. I live a different class of life. I'm down 3st 4lbs since I started. All is possible, just trust the process!

Danielle Kennedy (Galway)

I have struggled with my weight and, as a result, my self-esteem for over thirty years now. I was always a 'big' child and the 'plump' sister.

In my early twenties, I, like so many other women, joined a slimming club and attended for almost 16 years. I did manage to lose three stone TWICE but couldn't manage to keep it off, blaming my full-time job and three kids. This year I made the decision to try Pat's programme and started following his plan. Within weeks, I had family, friends, and colleagues, asking me if I had lost weight. My clothes started feeling looser, I had an abundance of energy, and my skin, hair and nails all benefited too. Now, fast approaching 40, I have never been stronger or fitter. I've probably been lighter but I've never been thinner! Thanks Pat.

Motivational Playlist as Suggested by the PDF Facebook Fans

I asked, you answered! Throughout the book, I will be featuring the tunes that help you stay motivated during your work outs!

1. **Macklemore – Can't Hold Us**
2. **Daft Punk – Harder Better Faster Stronger**
3. **Blur – Girls and Boys**
4. **Red Hot Chilli Peppers – Can't Stop**
5. **Florence and the Machine – Rabbit Heart**
6. **David Guetta Ft Nicki Minaj – Turn Me On**
7. **The Ting Tings – That's Not My Name**
8. **Vampire Weekend – A-Punk**
9. **N.E.R.D. – She Likes To Move**
10. **Jackson 5 – ABC**

FITNESS – THE TRUTH

CHAPTER 7

21 Day Jump Start – The Prep

> 'Don't hope you will succeed, know you will succeed.' – PAT DIVILLY

Step 1: Food

Food is going to account for the majority of your results, so rid your kitchen of any foods that are not compliant with your shopping list for the *21 Day Jump Start*. (Don't throw the food away, give it to a homeless shelter or a soup kitchen.) Willpower will only take you so far, but, if you clear the cupboards of any sugary junk, then you will be giving yourself a really strong opportunity to succeed. By all means, you can try following the plan while your kitchen is full of treats, but why make the process even more difficult than it has to be? If the chocolate isn't there, then you can't eat it! It really is as simple as that.

By getting rid of all the foods that are not working for you, you are not only setting yourself up for success, you are also confirming for yourself that you are serious about adopting this new and healthy lifestyle. Think about it. When you start this plan, you are literally refusing to be a victim of circumstance; you are refusing to spend another day complaining about your weight, or criticising yourself whenever you look in the mirror. You are taking responsibility. Don't just hope you will succeed, know you will succeed.

> 'Few people take objectives really seriously. They put average effort into too many things, rather than superior thought and effort into a few important things. People who achieve the most are selective as well as determined.' – RICHARD KOCH

You will be eating mainly fresh food, so you might find it necessary to do a grocery shop twice a week. If, however, you shop around then you should find plenty of bargains. Remember, not all healthy food has to be expensive. If you do your research first, you will find the products you want, for the best prices. Simple things like establishing a good relationship with your local butcher or green grocer may mean you can get good deals by being a regular customer.

PDF Tip

A teaspoon of coconut oil right off the spoon is good for combating sugar cravings.

The Shopping List

Here is a list of the permitted foods for the *21 Day Jump Start*. You don't need absolutely everything on this list; just choose the things you think you will enjoy.

Miscellaneous

✔ Coconut oil. (You need to be cooking everything in this! If, for some reason, you can't get your hands on it, then try using extra virgin olive oil instead.)

✔ Cashew nut and almond nut butter.

✔ Hummus.

✔ Full Greek style yogurt (or live yoghurt, unflavoured).

Beverages

✔ Water. (Bottled only. No tap water! Buy in bulk for convenience and affordability.)

✔ Green tea.

✔ Herbal and fruit teas.

✔ Tulsi tea.

✔ Black coffee.

✔ Almond, coconut, or, hazelnut milk.

Herbs/ Sauces/Spices

✔ Apple cider vinegar.
✔ Balsamic vinegar.
✔ Spices such as cinnamon, turmeric, paprika, chilli, etc.

✔ Sea salt.
✔ Lemon juice.
✔ Frank's Hot Sauce.
✔ Nandos peri peri (sauce, not marinade).

Meat/ Eggs/Poultry

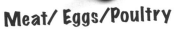

- ✔ Chicken, or, turkey breasts.
- ✔ Beef.
- ✔ Lamb.
- ✔ Duck.
- ✔ Free range eggs.

Fish/Seafood

- ✔ Cod.
- ✔ Fresh tuna.
- ✔ Mackerel.
- ✔ Salmon.
- ✔ Bass.
- ✔ Scallop.
- ✔ Trout.
- ✔ Lobster.

Vegetables

- ✔ Fresh OR frozen is fine. Dark green vegetables are best. The more you can eat of these, the better! Avoid parsnips and carrots however, unless you are looking to gain weight.

- ✔ Aubergine.
- ✔ Avocados.
- ✔ Beetroot.
- ✔ Basil.
- ✔ Broccoli.
- ✔ Cauliflower.
- ✔ Courgettes.
- ✔ Cucumber.
- ✔ Fresh parsley.
- ✔ Green beans.
- ✔ Kale.
- ✔ Lettuce (dark leaved).
- ✔ Onion.
- ✔ Peppers.
- ✔ Roasted veggies.
- ✔ Rocket.
- ✔ Spring onions.
- ✔ Spinach.
- ✔ Watercress.

Nuts

- ✔ Raw and unsalted, no peanuts!
- ✔ Almonds.
- ✔ Brazil nuts.
- ✔ Cashews.
- ✔ Chia seeds.
- ✔ Macadamias.
- ✔ Pecans.
- ✔ Pine nuts.
- ✔ Pistachios.
- ✔ Pumpkin seeds.
- ✔ Sesame seeds.
- ✔ Walnuts.
- ✔ Flax seeds.

Starchy Carbs

If weight loss is your primary goal, starchy carbs, such as those featured on the list here, are best avoided for the duration of the 21 days. These foods would be more suitable for those of you who are more active, or who might be looking to maintain their current weight. They are best taken at breakfast or post-workout. Check out Chapter 10 – Day 22 & Beyond, for information on how to carb cycle for continued fat loss and health.

- ✗ Quinoa.
- ✗ Brown basmati or brown long grain rice.
- ✗ Sweet potato.
- ✗ Rice noodles.
- ✗ Carrots.

Fruits

Like the starchy carbs, avoid these for the first 14 days if your primary goal is weight loss.

As you can see, there is no alcohol, gluten, dairy, or processed foods (with the odd exception) on the shopping list! You will effectively be detoxing for the first two weeks.

- ✗ Apples.
- ✗ Bananas.
- ✗ Berries.
- ✗ Lemons.
- ✗ Limes.
- ✗ Plums.
- ✗ Watermelon.
- ✗ Gluten free oatcakes.

How to Eat Out on the 21 Day Jump Start

People sometimes overcomplicate this part, but it's actually very simple and straightforward. Pick your protein source, (meat, fish, poultry) and make sure it's as close to its natural state as possible. That means nothing breaded or crumbed! Ask for any sauces to be kept on the side. If you need to add flavour, balsamic vinegar or olive oil are perfectly fine substitutes. Instead of chips or potatoes, just ask for double portions of vegetables or salad. For drinks, you can have herbal teas, coffee, or water. Tea is fine but no sugar is allowed! If you like to take milk in your tea, remember, dairy is completely out, so replace it with either almond milk, rice milk, or coconut milk. In terms of taste, rice milk is probably the closest substitute for dairy.

Healthy Alternatives For Bad Foods

Below are a list of the most commonly bought grocery items, and the foods that you can replace them with. No excuses!

Craving	Healthy Alternative
Milk (Dairy)	Rice milk /Almond milk /Coconut milk
Bread	Gluten free bread.
Butter (Dairy)	Almond butter
Milk chocolate	A square of good quality dark chocolate. Look for cocoa content over 70%.
Cheese	Goats cheese or feta (not from cow's milk)
Cereal	Gluten free porridge.
Fizzy Drinks	Coconut Water.
Ice Cream	Full Fat Greek Style yogurt with blueberries.
Salty Snacks	Unsalted nuts and seeds.

Try to change your outlook on the foods you used to crave. Don't view them as temptations, view them for what they are: the reason you are now unhappy with your weight.

Step 2: Supplements

Pay for the content, not the hype!

I would strongly advise that you shop around for your supplements. You will definitely pick up some great deals, particularly online. Good marketing will often lead people to believe that the more expensive brands are better than then cheaper ones. The reality, however, is that a lot of supplements from both ends of the price spectrum are actually made in the same factories. This is typically the case with the protein powders. The only real difference is that the more expensive brands are heavily marketed. The one supplement I would strongly encourage you to spend more a little money on, is fish oil. The quality of the oil is dependent on the levels of the two main active ingredients – EPA, and DHA. The higher the content of these two ingredients, the higher the price, so, with this in mind, it would be wise to invest in a good brand. For all your other supplement needs, however, you will definitely pick up some inexpensive 'white label brands', where you pay only for the content and not the hype.

PDF Weight Loss Tip

If you are eating a very 'clean' diet and not seeing the results you want, digestive health may be an issue. If your body isn't capable of properly digesting the foods you are taking in, then you will struggle to perform optimally. Digestive enzymes, glutamine, and pro-biotics are three supplements that can help improve gut health and digestion.

Step 3: Training Partner/Routine

You are about to embark upon a whole new transformation, so take a look at your circle of friends and ask yourself which ones will really support you throughout your journey, and which ones are likely to tempt you off track? You become a reflection of the people you spend most of your time with, so are you going to hang around with the people who discourage you, or the people who keep your fired up when your motivation levels run low? You can do this on your own, but why make life difficult for yourself? Make a firm decision to surround yourself only with like-minded people who will support you and keep you on track.

Once you have your food and supplements sorted, look at your training routine. Decide if you need a training partner; someone who is going to hold you accountable. Be specific when planning your workouts. Where are you going to train? When are you going to train? When can you set the necessary time aside to train? Treat your workout like you would an appointment. Little things are always going to come up, but you wouldn't cancel an appointment because a friend called around to the house for a chat, so try to afford the same degree of importance to your workouts. Make the *21 Day Jump Start* a priority. This is your goal, and one that will benefit you in so many ways, so don't stray from it.

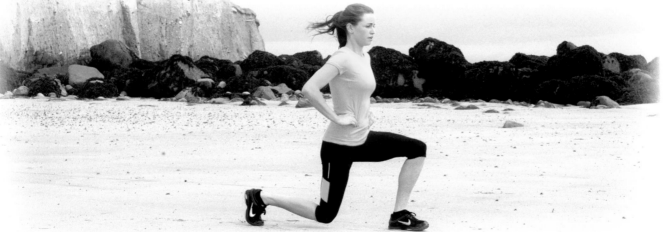

Step 4: Training Journal

Some people find it helpful to keep a written log of the process, from the food they eat, to the workouts they complete. Doing this allows them to look back on their hard work, and establish which workouts gave them the best and worst results. When it comes to goals, it's all about clarity. This is why a training journal can be so helpful. Once you have it on paper, there is no disputing it because it goes from being a daydream, to being a firm goal on paper. Use your training journal to log the time it took to complete your runs. Write down how many repetitions you did, how many squats you carried out and the times you did them in. This will give you a good baseline; something to improve upon the following week.

Best For Energy:

- Wheatgrass
- Super greens drink (which you will find in any health food shop)

If you are feeling tired and run down, chances are its because your body is in an acidic state. Counteract this problem by alkalising your body. Green drinks are one of the best ways to do this.

Step 5: Hydration

Hydration is a big part of the plan. Set yourself up for success by buying a crate of bottled water. Always have a few bottles of water in the car, and a bottle or two by the front door so you can grab one as you are leaving the house. If you don't like drinking just water, then you can add a squeeze of fresh lemon or lime to it. Keep snacks like nuts and seeds in the car or in the office. That way, on the days when you are caught up in traffic or in work, and can't get your next meal, the snacks will keep you from feeling hungry.

PDF Tip

When preparing dinner, try cooking a double portion. This will take care of your lunch for the following day as well.

Ideally, your goals should be both aesthetic and performance focused. Of course you want to look good, but if you work towards improving your performance, then the weight loss will take care of itself.

Instead of deciding that you want to lose ten pounds, maybe set your sights on running ten kilometres in a specific amount of time, or, signing up for your first race? Set yourself a goal and a deadline, but make both of them measurable. It's pointless to say, 'I want to lose weight'. You have to be specific. Once you establish clarity on your dream, it immediately becomes an achievable goal.

The Prep Checklist

1. Is my kitchen filled only with foods that are compliant with the 21 Day plan?
2. Have I set aside a specific amount of time each day for my workout?
3. Do I need a training partner?
4. Do I have all of the necessary supplements?
5. Am I surrounding myself with people who will bring me down, or lift me higher?
6. Do I have a training journal?
7. Have I set specific goals and deadlines?
8. Have I put snacks and bottles of water on my desk at work, in the car, by the front door, etc?

PDF Tip

Shift work

If you work shifts, you can still accurately follow the *21 Day Jump Start*. Everything remains the same. You just need to ensure that you maximise the quality of the sleep you do get. Make sure your room is pitch dark, turn off all electronic devices and artificial lights in the room.

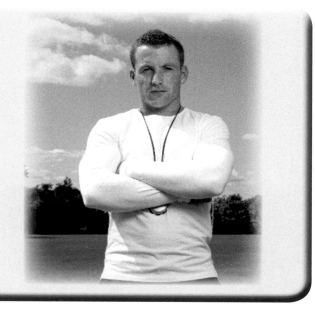

Nora Napier (Mayo)

Discovering Pat Divilly Fitness is definitely one of the best things that has ever happened me. I have done plenty of diets in my life, but that's what they were, diets. They weren't doable in the long term.

What Pat has passed on to me will stick with me for life. I have suffered with migraines since I was a child. Since implementing what Pat has taught me I haven't had one. I used to be a bad sleeper, I was bloated and was just unmotivated. I now sleep better, have way more energy and my skin has improved. I even like most vegetables now, lots of which I wouldn't even try before, and I find myself more experimental when cooking and trying different dishes. I took part in my first mini marathon (the first of many, hopefully) a couple of weeks ago, I've also taken part in a few 5k events. I intend climbing Croagh Patrick in the very near future too. I would never have

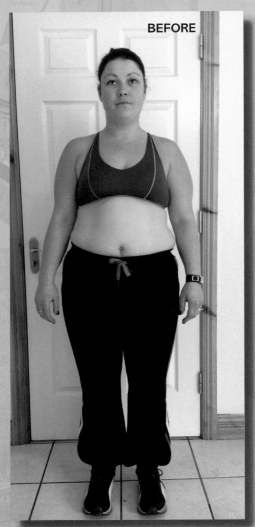
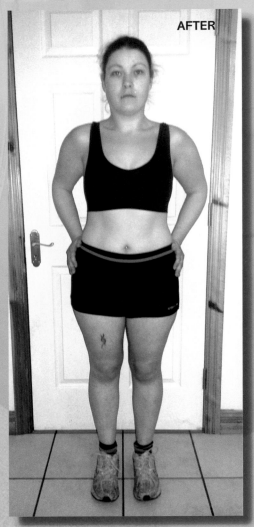

BEFORE

AFTER

been able to do any of these things before as I was so unfit. I'd be puffed out walking to the neighbours' house. I now find that I look forward to my workout. It really sets me up for the day and if there's a day that I cannot do it I feel crap. I was always a scales watcher, but I've learned that the numbers on the scales don't mean much. It's the inch loss and how you feel in your clothes that matter most. They are ultimately the biggest signs that you're becoming leaner. I am still a work in progress, but, to date, I have lost 38 inches. I'm still working on it. I am so grateful for all the knowledge that Pat has passed on to me. I'm just sorry I didn't find him sooner. Everyone would benefit from this man's knowledge. He is going to change the health of the nation and further. Thanks Pat for all your help in achieving my goals!

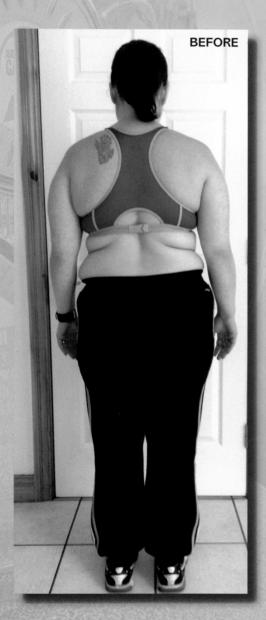
BEFORE

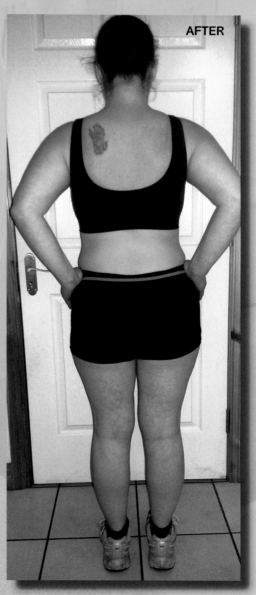
AFTER

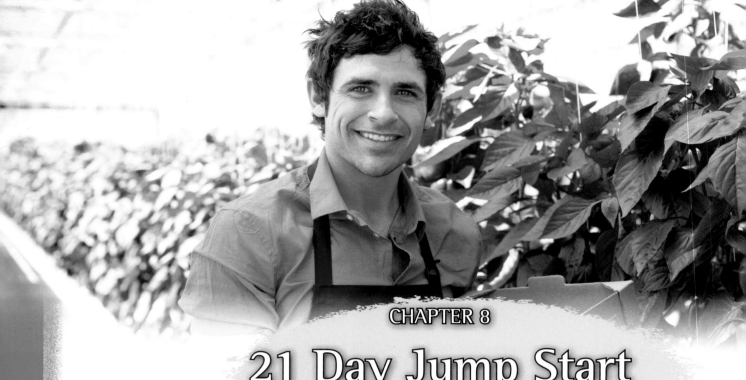

CHAPTER 8

21 Day Jump Start
- The Plan

Detox Symptoms: What to Expect, and When They Will Pass

During the first couple of days of this plan, you can expect to experience detox-like symptoms. Your body holds toxins in your fat cells, so in order to release those toxins, they have to return to the blood stream first. This is precisely why you get those typical detox symptoms such as low energy and headaches. Some people even report getting a slight rash, but this is just a sign of the toxins leaving the body through the skin. Those symptoms pass after three or four days, and it's following this time frame that you will start to feel and enjoy your natural energy. By the end of week one, people should feel a noticeable surge of energy. You are wide awake in the morning when you get up, your quality of sleep is better. The detox symptoms should not go past day four. The sugar cravings may take a little longer, depending on how reliant the person has been on sugar. You should notice the cravings fading somewhat as you enter week two.

Hunger Pangs: You Won't Get Them!

Don't fret over the prospect of suffering from pangs of hunger. These won't happen because your intake of healthy fats will have suppressed your appetite. The mistake a lot of people make is that when they cut back on the sugar, they don't replace it with anything. When you cut sugar from your daily diet, yes you will be cutting out a massive amount of calories, but this isn't the right approach. Keep the calorie count around the same, but instead, aim to take in a better quality of calorie. For instance, when you decrease your intake of sugar, increase your intake of healthy fats. You are simply replacing a bad, weight gaining calorie with a good calorie that won't cause you to gain weight!

Meal Plans: Be Creative!

The dishes featured in the *21 Day Jump Start* are just examples of what you can create with the foods allowed in this plan, so don't freak out and assume you have to buy everything I have mentioned. Play around with the ingredients and create dishes more to your liking if you wish. The important thing is that you structure your meals to include a protein source, a fat source, and plenty of greens.

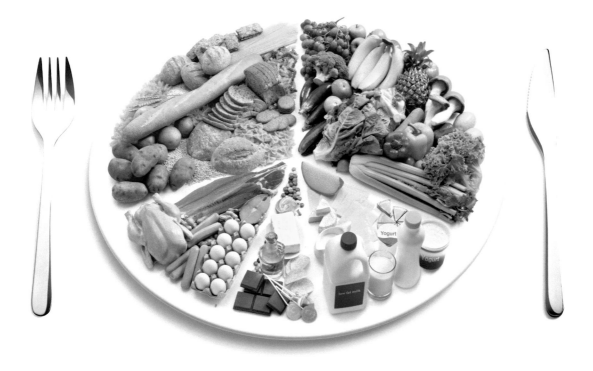

S

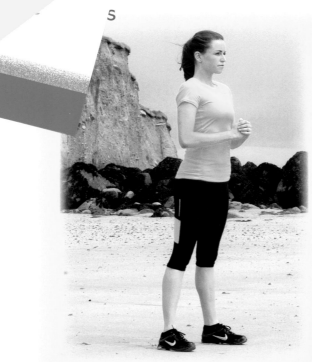

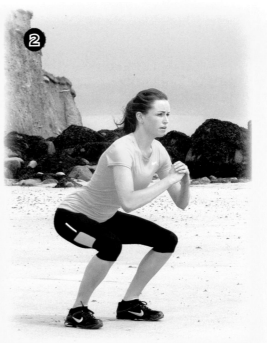

Starting with your feet shoulder width apart sit back as if sitting into a chair.

Ensure you keep your chest up throughout and heels on the floor. Once your hips are as low as your knees stand back up to your start position.

SQUAT JUMPS

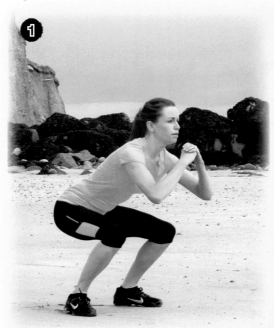

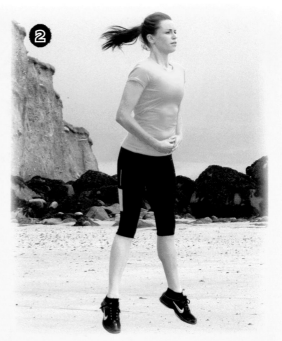

If you are already comfortable with the regular squat you can add a little jump for a tougher progression.

Instead of returning to the standing position, jump and land softly back into the squat. Again, be sure to keep the weight on your heels, your chest big throughout.

LUNGES

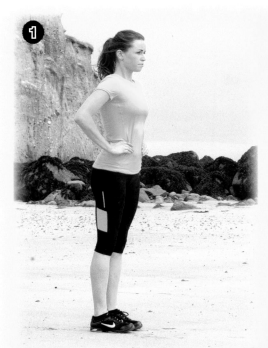

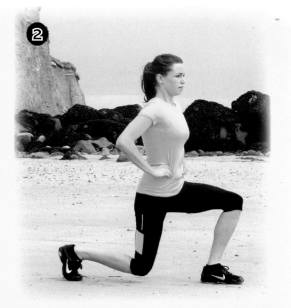

With hands on your hips and standing tall, take a big step forward with one leg. Lower your hips until your back knee is almost touching the floor.

Push off your front leg bringing it back to your start position. Remember when stepping to take a big enough step that your knee doesn't come over your toe. Your shin should be in a straight line at the bottom of the lunge.

KNEE DRIVE

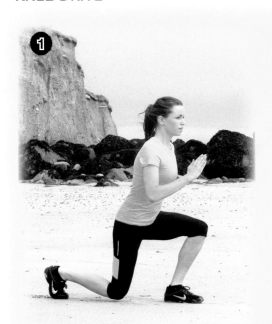

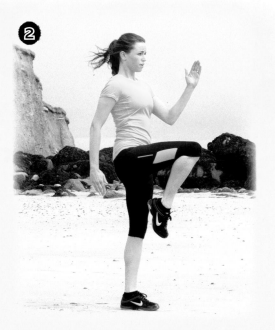

This is a progression to the lunge that will test your balance a little. Instead of stepping forward take a big step back lowering the moving knee toward the floor.

Now instead of stopping at the start position when returning the leg, drive the knee forward and pause for a second keeping your balance.

STEP UPS

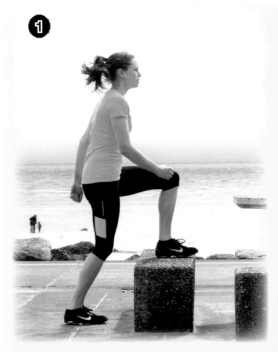

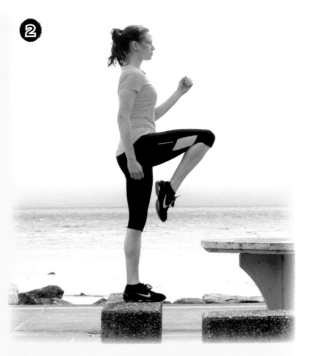

Standing tall, step with one leg onto a bench, chair or step that is just below knee level.

Bring your other knee up and pause for a second before returning both feet to the floor. Take your time!

PUSH UPS

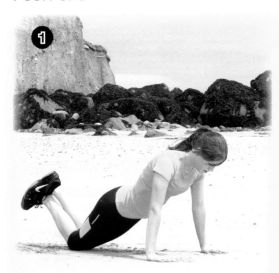

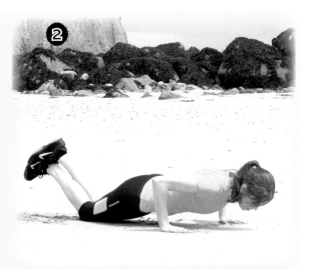

Starting with your knees on the floor, a straight line from your knee to your shoulder and your hands over your shoulders, lower your chest slowly toward the floor.

Your elbows should now be bent. Extend your arms to return to the start position.

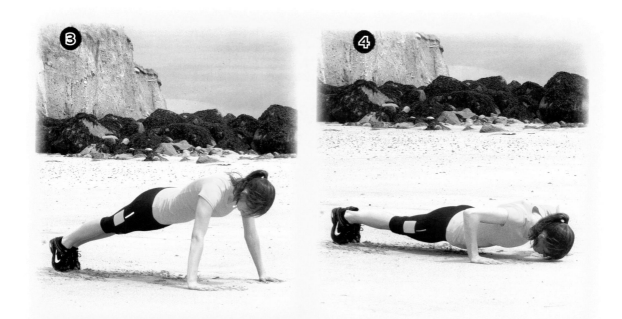

If the push up with knees on the floor is too easy, then you can perform the same movement with feet on the floor and knees elevated.

BURPEES

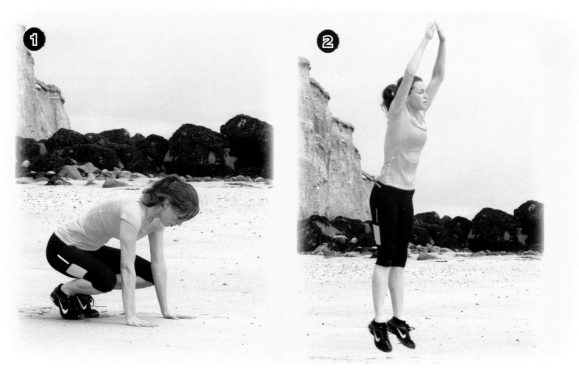

Starting from standing place your hands to the floor. Kick your feet back so that you are in the push up position.

Kick the feet forward again before returning to standing. Finish with a jump and hands reached overhead.

MOUNTAIN CLIMBERS

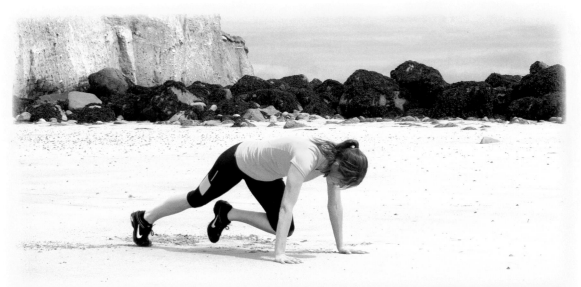

Starting from the press up position tuck one knee toward your chest. Bring that knee back and the other forward switching back and forth. Take your time until you have found a rhythm.

HIP BRIDGES

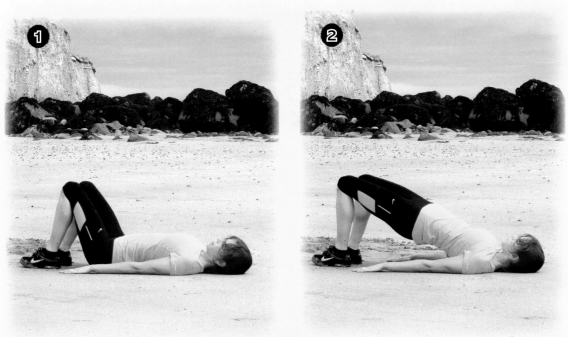

Starting on your back with your feet flat on the floor, around shoulder width apart.

Push your hips toward the ceiling and squeeze your bum tight for 2-3 seconds before slowly lowering to the start position.

21 DAY JUMP START

PLANKS

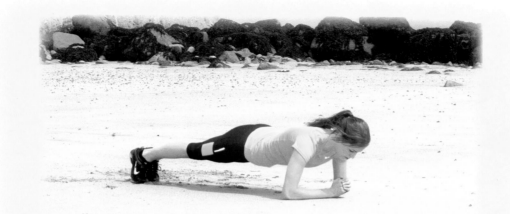

Starting in the position shown with feet and elbows on the floor and a straight line from your heal to your shoulder. You should have your thumbs under your nose. Don't allow your hips to come too high or drop low. Maintain the straight line.

SIDE PLANKS

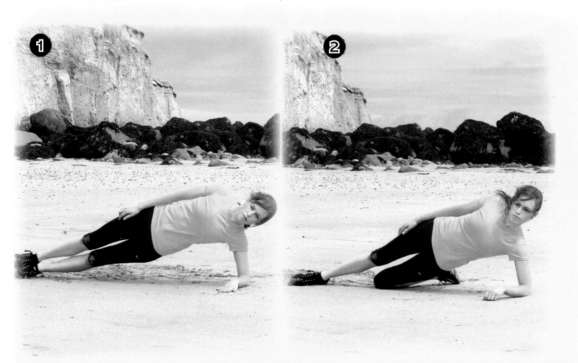

Starting on your side in the position shown, rest your weight on your elbow and feet and elevate your hips as high as you can. Hold this position for the allotted time.

If you cannot perform the movement with both feet on the floor an easier version can be performed by placing your bottom knee down. You should still be looking to elevate your hips as much as you can from this position.

STRETCHES

QUADRICEP STRETCH

Can be performed standing or lying. Kick your foot to your bum to stretch the quadricep (large muscle at front of the leg). If standing raise your opposite arm straight in the air to get a stretch down your side. Hold for 15-30 seconds before repeating on the other leg.

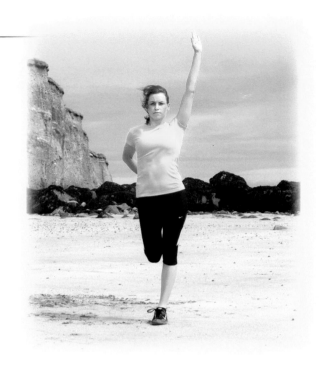

HAMSTRING STRETCH

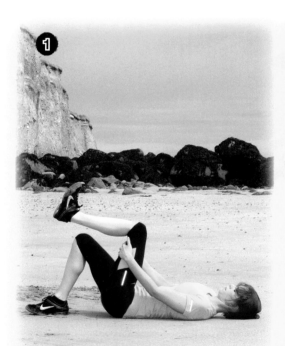

Lying on your back with your feet flat on the floor, hug the back of one of your knees and pull it toward your stomach.

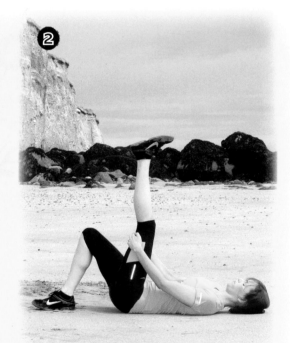

To stretch the hamstring straighten out your leg and point your toes toward your shin. Hold for around 30 seconds before repeating on the other leg.

COBRA/CAT STRETCH

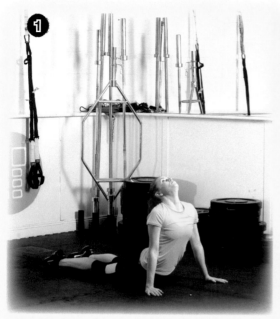

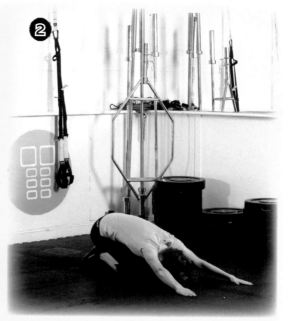

Lying on your front with hips low to the floor and hands flat on the floor look up toward the ceiling stretching the back.

Hold for around 15-30 seconds before sitting back to the 'cat stretch' again holding for 15-30 seconds.

Motivational Playlist as Suggested by the PDF Facebook Fans

1. **Blade – Vampire Dance Club Theme**
2. **50 cent – Ready For War**
3. **Avicii – 'Levels' Skrillex Remix**
4. **The Stooges – Push It Like A Dog (Soulwax Remix)**
5. **Felix Da Housecat – Silver**
6. **Macklemore – Thrift Shop**
7. **Gossip – Standing In The Way Of Control**
8. **The Yeah Yeah Yeahs – Heads Will Roll**
9. **Eminem – I'm Not Afraid**
10. **Prodigy – Omen**

Assessment Day

If you skip this step, I promise you, you will regret it!

The day before you begin the *21 Day Jump Start*, take three photographs and record your measurements. Repeat the process on day 21. By comparing the before and after pics, you will be able to see how much your body has changed in 21 days. This method will allow you to accurately track your progress. Far too many people are fixated by the scales, but the most important gauge of your progress is how you look in the mirror, how you feel on a day to day basis, and how you move in you workouts and every day life. You may not notice the subtle changes taking place to your body every day, but when you look back at your before pictures on day 21, you will realise just how far you have come.

Take the following three starting photos. (Make sure you are photographed full length and against a plain background.)

1. Front view, facing the camera.
2. Back view, with your back to the camera.
3. Side view, with one side to the camera.

As well as the photos, I would like you to take the following measurements (in inches).

Weight:	Stones and pounds on weight scale.
Waist:	Measurement around your belly button.
Chest:	Women, measure under the bust. Men, measure around the nipple.
Hips:	The top of your hips.
Waist:	Around your belly button.
Upper Leg:	At its widest point.
Arms:	From the middle of the bicep.

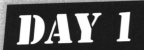

mon

DAY 1

Take it at your own pace today. If fat loss is your primary goal then diet will contribute to a lot of your results. If you get the diet spot on, you are over half way there so just focus on easing yourself into the fitness routine and take your time familiarising yourself with them. There's no point injuring yourself.

Meal Plan

Breakfast: *Two scrambled eggs with smoked salmon, asparagus, and goats cheese.*

Snack: *Handful of raspberries.*

Lunch: *Chicken and avocado salad with mixed greens and walnuts.*

Dinner: *Cod with stir fry vegetables cooked in coconut oil.*

Snack: *Small serving of Brazil nuts (6-12).*

DAY 1 WORKOUT:
UPPER BODY, CORE AND CARDIO!

Warm Up

Push Ups: 5 sets of 10 repetitions. Take 45 seconds break between each set. Pick the variation that is most suitable for you. Beginners should go with knees on the floor, more advanced trainees with knees off the floor. Take your time. This week is about familiarising yourself with the exercises.

Planks: 5 sets of 30-60 second holds. Hold the plank position for as long as you can, with good form, working up to holding for a full minute. Repeat for 5 sets taking 45 seconds break between sets.

Mountain Climbers: 4 sets of 30 seconds repetitions. Perform 30 seconds of mountain climbers followed by a 30 second break. Repeat for 4 sets.

Hip Bridges: 5 sets of 10 repetitions. Perform 5 sets of 10 repetitions taking 45 seconds rest between each set.

20 minute cardio block: Complete a 20 minute walk, jog or run (this is relative to your current fitness level). Your goal is to cover as much distance as you can in the 20 minute block. Keep track of the distance you cover. This will be important over the course of the programme.

Cool down!

DAY 2

There's a good chance you are experiencing some soreness today as a result of yesterday's work out. Don't panic! It's just a sign that your body is adjusting to the new routine. Focus on good hydration and keeping the nutrition clean. Stretching and hydration are the main solutions, but, if you are particularly sore, then take an Epsom salt bath.

Meal Plan

Breakfast: Chicken breast served with green beans and flaked almonds.

Snack: Can of tinned salmon.

Lunch: Turkey salad with 100g turkey, mixed greens, tomato, avocado and balsamic vinegar.

Dinner: *AJ's Turkey burger served with watercress, spinach and kale.

Snack: 100g full fat Greek style yogurt and blueberries

DAY 2 WORKOUT: LEGS

Warm Up

Squats: 5 sets of 10 repetitions. 5 sets of squats taking 45 seconds break between each set. Remember you are looking to get your hips as low as your knees on every repetition! Make sure you are keeping your heals on the floor and chest up throughout.

Lunges: 5 sets of 10 (each leg). Alternating legs, perform 10 repetitions off each leg before taking a 45 second break. Remember to keep good posture throughout and take big steps. Your back knee should almost touch the floor on each repetition.

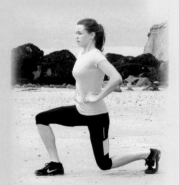

Step Ups: 4 sets of 8 repetitions (each leg). Perform 8 repetitions on your left leg before switching to your right leg. Take 45 seconds rest and repeat for 4 sets.

Hip Bridges: 5 sets of 10 repetitions. Perform 5 sets of 10 repetitions taking 45 seconds rest between each set. Focus on really squeezing the glutes at the top of the movement. Take your time with these!

High Knees: 5 sets of 30 seconds. Perform 30 seconds of high knees jogging on the spot followed by a 30 second break. Repeat for 5 sets!

Cool down!

* See recipe on page 101

'Believe that you can do it and you're halfway there!'

DAY 3

You might be experiencing detox-like symptoms today. In order for toxins to leave the body, they have to re-enter the blood stream, and this is why you are most likely feeling a bit crappy today. The headaches and low energy levels will have passed by Day 4 or 5 at latest. Stick it out! Once the toxins are out, you will enjoy a surge of natural energy and you will feel ten times better. Stay well hydrated and make sure you are eating plenty of good fats to replace the sugar you have ditched from your diet.

DAY 3 WORKOUT:
ACTIVE RECOVERY!

Today is your first active recovery day. I just want you to get out for a 40 minute brisk walk or slow jog.

'When you feel like giving up, remember why you started!'

Meal Plan

Breakfast: Two poached eggs, turkey bacon and two grilled tomatoes.

Snack: 100g full fat Greek style yogurt with cinnamon.

Lunch: Grilled chicken breast with mixed vegetables.

Dinner: Cod fillet served with green beans.

Snack: Small serving macadamia nuts (6-12).

'The trick is to enjoy life. Don't wish away your days, waiting for better ones ahead.'
— MARJORIE PAY HINCKLEY

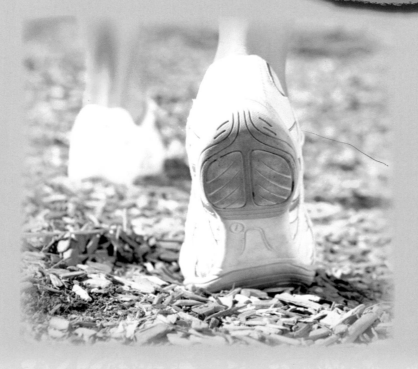

DAY 4

Remember, the worse you are during the detox phase, the more you need it! The same applies to your workouts. The more achey you are following a work out, the more your body needs it.

DAY 4 WORKOUT: UPPER BODY, CORE AND CARDIO!

Warm Up

Push Ups: 5 sets of 10 repetitions. Take 45 seconds break between each set. Pick the variation that is most suitable for you. Beginners should go with knees on the floor, more advanced trainees with knees off the floor and very strong trainees with feet elevated on a chair or step.

Planks: 5 sets of 30-60 second holds. Hold the plank position for as long as you can with good form working up to holding for a full minute. Repeat for 5 sets taking 45 seconds break between sets.

Mountain Climbers: 4 sets of 30 seconds repetitions. Perform 30 seconds of mountain climbers followed by a 30 second break. Repeat for 4 sets.

Hip Bridges: 5 sets of 10 repetitions. Perform 5 sets of 10 repetitions taking 45 seconds rest between each set.

20 minute cardio block: Complete a 20 minute walk, jog or run (this is relative to your current fitness level). Your goal is to cover as much distance as you can in the 20 minute block. Keep track of the distance you cover. This will be important over the course of the programme.

Cool down!

* See recipe on page 96

** See recipe on page 98.

Meal Plan

Breakfast: *Divilly's Berry Blast Smoothie

Snack: Celery sticks dipped in two tablespoons cashew nut butter.

Lunch: **37 West Muscle Builder salad.

Dinner: Lamb skewers served with peppers and a mixed green salad.

Snack: 100g cottage cheese.

'Don't spend the rest of your life wondering if you can do it, start now!'

DAY 5

DAY 5 WORKOUT: LEGS!

Warm Up

Squats: 5 sets of 10 repetitions. 5 sets of squats taking 45 seconds break between each set. Remember you are looking to get your hips as low as your knees on every repetition! Make sure you are keeping your heals on the floor and chest up throughout.

Lunges: 5 sets of 10 (each leg). Alternating legs perform 10 repetitions off each leg before taking a 45 second break. Remember to keep good posture throughout and take big steps. Your back knee should almost touch the floor on each repetition.

Step Ups: 4 sets of 8 repetitions (each leg). Perform 8 repetitions on your left leg before switching to your right leg. Take 45 seconds rest and repeat for 4 sets.

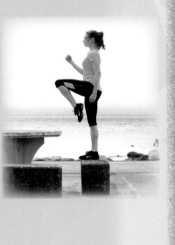

Hip Bridges: 5 sets of 10 repetitions. Perform 5 sets of 10 repetitions taking 45 seconds rest between each set. Focus on really squeezing the glutes at the top of the movement. Take your time with these!

High Knees: 5 sets of 30 seconds. Perform 30 seconds of high knees jogging on the spot followed by a 30 second break. Repeat for 5 sets!

Cool down!

> ### Meal Plan
> **Breakfast:** Bell pepper stuffed with turkey mince.
> **Snack:** Half an avocado.
> **Lunch:** Prawn salad.
> **Dinner:** Beef burger served with salad.
> **Snack:** Carrot sticks with two tablespoons of homemade hummus.

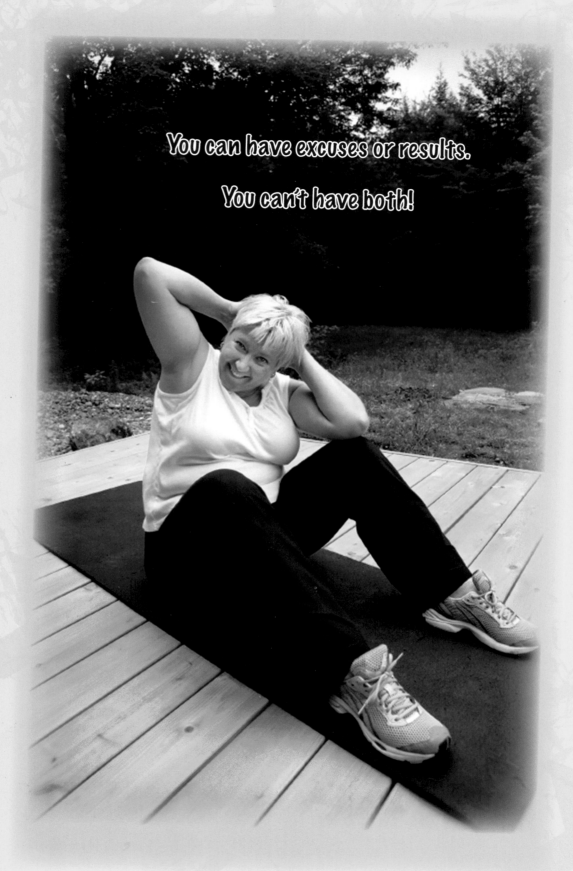

You can have excuses or results.

You can't have both!

DAYS 6 & 7

DAYS 6 AND 7 WORKOUTS: ACTIVE RECOVERY!

First weekend on the plan! We don't have any structured training but try to get out and about for at least 40 minutes of exercise on both days. This can be anything from a leisurely walk to a game of tennis or tag rugby with family or friends!

Plan out your weekend and don't let slip ups in the kitchen (or out on the town!) undo all your hard work from your first 5 days!

Meal Plan

Breakfast: *Three egg omelette with red onion, jalapenos and peppers.*

Snack: *Small serving of cashew nuts (8-12).*

Lunch: *Chicken and feta cheese salad.*

Dinner: *Baked cod with lemon, green beans and flaked almonds.*

Snack: *100g cottage cheese.*

Motivational Playlist as Suggested by the PDF Facebook Fans

1. **Avicii – Hey Brother**
2. **David Guetta – Play Hard**
3. **Kanye West – Mercy**
4. **NERD – She Wants To Move**
5. **Kanye West – The New Workout Plan (Short Version)**
6. **Gossip – Move In The Right Direction**
7. **Kelly Clarkson – What Doesn't Kill You Makes You Stronger**
8. **Foo Fighters – All My Life**
9. **Ride on time – Black box**
10. **Bastille – Pompeii (Kat Krazy remix)**

DAY 7

You know by now that preparation is key to the whole plan so take some time today to organise yourself for the upcoming week. The first week might have felt like it was dragging a bit because you were getting used to this new dramatic change, but every day of this plan is going to fly by so make every workout and meal count. The 21 days are going to pass whether you do this plan or not so you might as well do the plan and reap the rewards by the end of it.

Meal Plan

Breakfast: *Smoked salmon served on a bed of greens.*

Snack: *Celery sticks dipped in two tablespoons almond nut butter.*

Lunch: **37 West Superfood Salad.*

Dinner: *Beef burger (no bun) with steamed broccoli and spinach.*

Snack: *Hard boiled egg.*

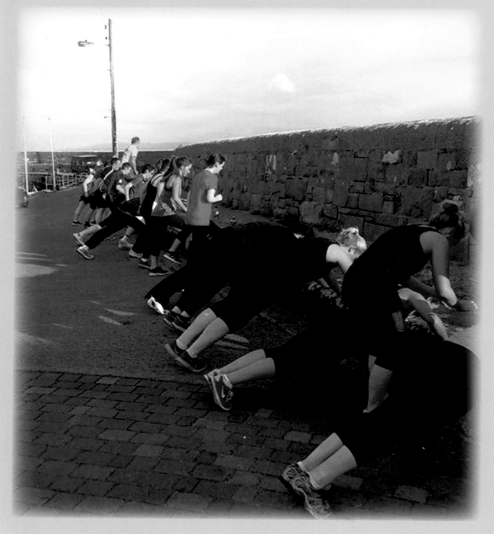

* See recipe on page 98.

DAY 8

You should be very familiar with the exercise movements by now, so increase the intensity from today onwards. Even if you try to improve each exercise by 1%, it will pay off. Remember the compound effect I told you about earlier in the book! Your progress doesn't need to happen in massive leaps, it just needs to be consistent.

Meal Plan

Breakfast: *Turkey slices and a small handful of almonds.*

Snack: *Handful of blueberries.*

Lunch: *Tuna salad.*

Dinner: *Cod fillet with steamed vegetables.*

Snack: *Small serving of brazil nuts (8-12).*

DAY 8 WORKOUT:
INTERVAL TRAINING!

Warm up.

Squats: 5 sets of 40 seconds work, 20 seconds break. Here you will use an interval timer or stop watch to track 40 seconds of work where you perform as many squats as you can with good form. Take a 20 second break before repeating for a total of 5 sets. Try to count your repetitions in your first 40 second set and maintain that number for the following 5 sets! After 5 sets, take a 60-90 second break.

Knee Drives: 4 sets of 40 seconds work, 20 second break. Start with your left leg stepping back and knee then driving forward and perform as many repetitions as you can in 40 seconds. Take a 20 second break before repeating with your right leg. Once you have performed 4 sets (two off of each leg) take a 60-90 second break before moving to push ups.

Push Ups: 4 sets of 40 seconds work, 20 seconds break. Perform as many push ups as you can in 40 seconds followed by a 20 second break. Repeat for 4 sets before taking a minute long break. Stick with whichever push up variation you are comfortable with.

Plank: 5 sets of 40 seconds work, 20 seconds break. Perform 5 sets of the plank looking to hold for 40 seconds followed by a 20 second break. Take one minute to rest after 5 sets. If the plank is a new exercise for you, a 40 second hold may be a struggle. Look to work up to this.

Jump Squats: 3 sets of 30 seconds work, 30 seconds break. Perform as many jump squats as you can with good form in 30 seconds before taking a 30 second break. Repeat for 3 sets. Focus on landing softly back into the squat! (If you aren't comfortable with jump squats you can stick with regular squats here).

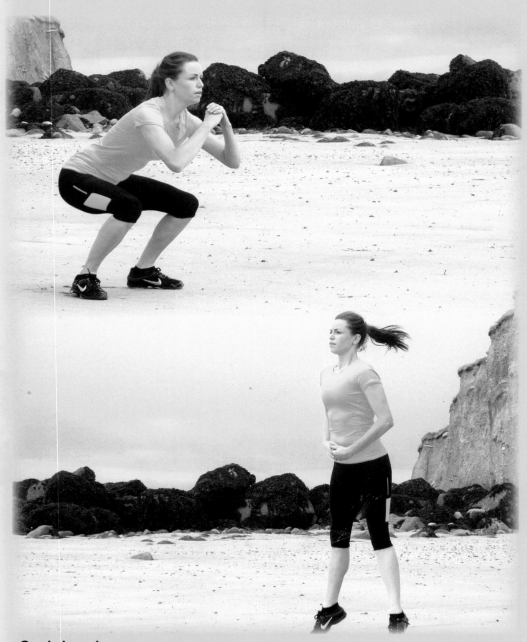

Cool down!

DAY 9

'Tell your heart that the fear of suffering is worse than the suffering itself. And no heart has ever suffered when it goes in search of its dream'.

- PAULO COELHO

Meal Plan

Breakfast: Chicken breast and a handful of walnuts.

Snack: Carrots and celery sticks with *Galway guacamole.

Lunch: Turkey salad with 100g of turkey, mixed greens, tomato, avocado and balsamic vinegar.

Dinner: Roast beef with steamed veggies.

Snack: Tin of tuna.

DAY 9 WORKOUT:
TIME TRIAL!

Warm up.

Today you've got a 30 minute walk, jog or run looking to cover as much distance as possible! Regardless of your fitness level this should test you. Use a Smart Phone app, a running track, or a familiar route, to ensure you can get an accurate gauge of the distance you have covered.

Keep track of your distance covered, you'll need this later in the programme!

Finish your session with some stretches to ensure you stay injury-free and mobile!

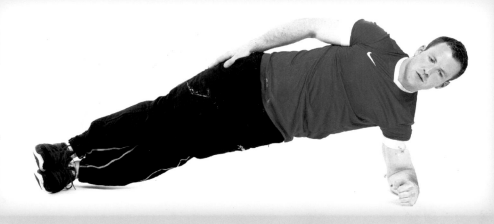

* See recipe on page 99.

DAY 10

DAY 10 WORKOUT: INTERVAL TRAINING!

Warm up.

Squats: 5 sets of 45 seconds work, 15 seconds break. Just like Monday's session but we will be going with 45 seconds of work followed by a 15 second break. After 5 sets take a 60-90 second rest.

Lunges: 4 sets of 45 seconds work, 15 second break. Alternating legs, perform lunges for 45 seconds before taking a 15 second break. Repeat for 4 sets before taking a 60 second break.

Push Ups: 4 sets of 45 seconds work, 15 seconds break. Perform as many push ups as you can in 40 seconds followed by a 20 second break. Repeat for 4 sets before taking a minute long break. Stick with whichever push up variation you are comfortable with.

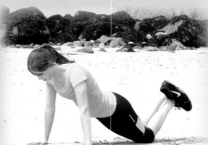

Side planks: 5 sets of 30 seconds left, 30 seconds right. Perform 5 sets of the side plank off of each side switching back and forth with no rest. 30 seconds off of your left side, 30 seconds off of your right side. Focus on keeping your hips as high as you can.

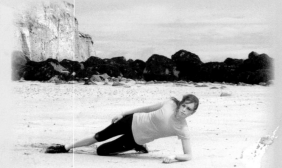

Mountain Climbers: 3 sets of 30 seconds work, 30 seconds break. 30 seconds of mountain climbers followed by 30 seconds of rest, repeated 3 times to finish out today's session!

Cool Down.

Meal Plan

Breakfast: Scrambled eggs with turkey bacon, grilled tomatoes and mushrooms.

Snack: 100g full fat Greek style yogurt with a scoop of protein powder.

Lunch: Grilled chicken breast with cauliflower mash.

Dinner: Steak with steamed green veggies.

Snack: Tin of salmon.

DAY 11

DAY 11 WORKOUT:
5KM AND CORE!

Warm Up.

Today you've got a 5km. I want you to complete this as quickly as you possibly can! Now, this is completely individual. You may need to walk the whole thing or you might be breaking records with your 5km time! Whatever your level, keep track of the time it takes you and get that time down on paper to have for later on in the programme. After your 5km run take a 3-5 minute break.

Next you have 5 sets of the 'Plank' with 60 seconds break between each set. Aim to hold for as close to a minute on each set as you can.

Finish the session with a cool down and stretches.

Meal Plan

Breakfast: *Rising Stars breakfast Smoothie.

Snack: Hard boiled egg.

Lunch: Steak with steamed veggies (dinner leftover from day 10).

Dinner: Sea bass served with asparagus and flaked almonds.

Snack: 100g cottage cheese.

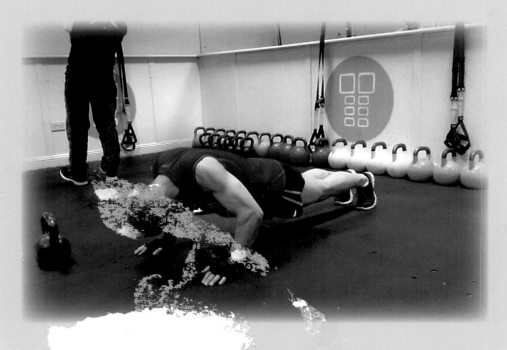

* See reci

DAY 12 WORKOUT:
INTERVAL TRAINING!

Warm Up.

Lunges: 5 sets of 40 seconds work, 20 seconds break. Alternating legs, perform lunges for 40 seconds before taking a 20 second break. Repeat for 5 sets before taking a 60 second rest.

Mountain Climbers: 4 sets of 40 seconds work, 20 second break. Perform mountain climbers for 40 seconds followed by a 20 second break. Repeat for 4 rounds.

Push Ups: 4 sets of 40 seconds work 20 seconds break. Perform as many push ups as you can in 40 seconds followed by a 20 second break. Repeat for 4 sets before taking a minute long break. Stick with whichever push up variation you are comfortable with.

Hip Bridges: 4 sets of 40 seconds work, 20 seconds break. Perform 40 seconds of hip bridges before taking 20 seconds rest. Repeat for 4 sets. Don't rush there, take your time and focus on good technique with a big squeeze of the glutes at the top!

Burpees: 3 sets of 40 seconds work, 20 seconds break. These are tough, but an excellent exercise! Perform burpees for 40 seconds followed by a 20 second break. Repeat for 3 rounds! Try to get as many repetitions in the second and third sets as you do the first.

Cool down!

Meal Plan

Breakfast: Bell pepper stuffed with beef mince.

Snack: Half an avocado.

Lunch: *Soup

Dinner: Thai green curry.

Snack: Carrots sticks with two tablespoons of homemade hummus

* See recipe on page 100.

DAY 13

DAYS 13 AND 14 WORKOUTS: ACTIVE RECOVERY!

Second weekend of the plan! Stay focused and try to get out for a 40 minute walk on both days.

Meal Plan

Breakfast: *Silver Strand Pina Colada Smoothie.

Snack: Small serving of cashew nuts (8-12).

Lunch: **Soup

Dinner: ***'Clean' Bolognese

Snack: Small handful of pumpkin or sesame seeds.

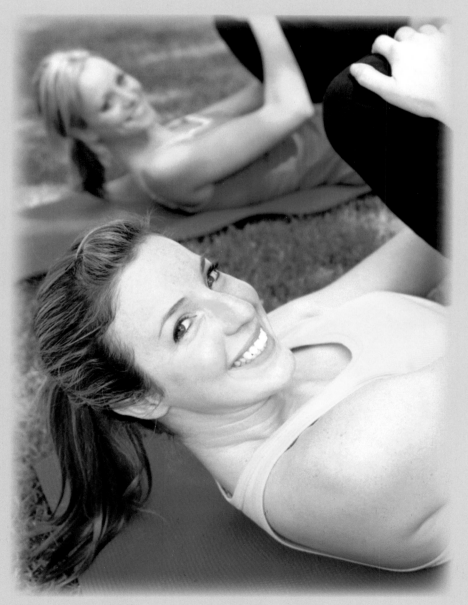

* See recipe on page 97.
** See recipe on page 100.
*** See recipe on page 102.

DAY 14

Two weeks in already! You should definitely be starting to see some results by now.

Meal Plan

Breakfast: Scrambled eggs with turkey bacon, grilled tomatoes and mushrooms.

Snack: Chicken breast.

Lunch: Egg salad.

Dinner: Steak fillet with mixed green salad or steamed vegetables.

Snack: Hard boiled egg.

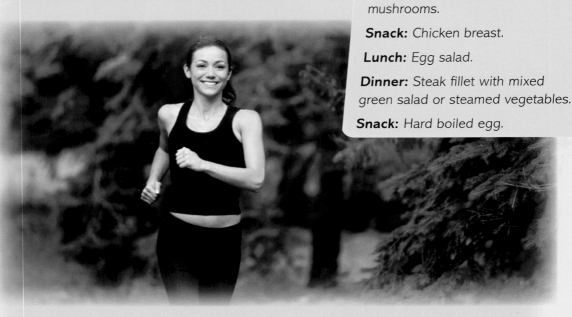

Motivational Playlist as Suggested by the PDF Facebook Fans

1. **The Prodigy – Breathe**
2. **Rudimental – Feel The Love**
3. **The entire Daft Punk Alive 2007 album!**
4. **Eminem – 'til I collapse**
5. **Bon Jovi – It's My Life**
6. **Rob Bailey and the Hustle Standard – Hungry**
7. **Katy Perry – Firework**
8. **Bon Jovi – Living On A Prayer**
9. **The Script – Hall Of Fame**
10. **WhiteSnake – Here I Go Again On My Own**

DAY 15

You are entering the final week of the plan so push yourself as much as possible. Increase the intensity again this week. Training is becoming more and more important as you become adjusted to your new diet. When you finish your last 5k run this week, consult with your previous times to see if you have improved on this.

DAY 15 WORKOUT: INTRODUCING 'THE FINISHER'!

Warm up.

Push Ups: 5 sets of 10 repetitions. Take 45 seconds break between each set. Pick the variation that is most suitable for you. Beginners should go with knees on the floor, more advanced trainees with knees off the floor. Take your time. This week is about familiarising yourself with the exercises.

Planks: 5 sets of 30-60 second holds. Hold the plank position for as long as you can with good form working up to holding for a full minute. Repeat for 5 sets taking 45 seconds break between sets.

Mountain Climbers: 4 sets of 30 seconds repetitions. Perform 30 seconds of mountain climbers followed by a 30 second break. Repeat for 4 sets.

Squats: 5 sets of 40 seconds work, 20 seconds break. Next you've got squats performed in your intervals of 40 seconds work, 20 seconds break for 5 sets. Take 60-90 seconds rest after completing the 5 sets.

10 minute 'Finisher': Today is the first day throwing in a 'finisher'. I'd like you to set a 10 minute countdown timer and perform the following sequence as many times as you can in the ten minutes:
- 10 Squats (or jump squats),
- 10 Push ups,
- 5 Burpees.

Every time you complete a circuit that is one round. See how many rounds you can complete in ten minutes with minimal rest between sets.

Cool down!

* See recipe on page 96.
** See recipe on page 98.

DAY 16

DAY 16 WORKOUT: REVISITING THE TIME TRIAL!

Going back to the time trial from day 9, you will be completing a 30 minute walk, jog or run looking to cover as much distance as possible. Before starting, look back at how much distance you covered in the time trial on day 9. Your goal for the day is to beat the distance covered by as much as possible!

Finish your session with some stretches and give yourself a pat on the back! I've no doubt you covered a little more distance today than you did on day 9. We talked about the compound effect earlier in the book. Small improvements on a daily basis lead to massive changes over time!

Meal Plan

Breakfast: Chicken breast and a handful of walnuts.

Snack: Carrots and celery sticks with *Galway guacamole.

Lunch: Ginger chicken lettuce cups.

Dinner: Cod fillet with steamed vegetables.

Snack: Tin of tuna.

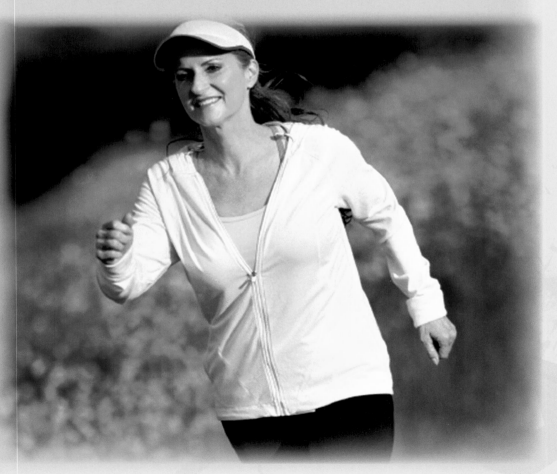

* See recipe on page 99.

DAY 17

DAY 17 WORKOUT: ANOTHER 'FINISHER'!

Warm Up.

Squats: 5 sets of 15 repetitions. Your legs should be getting stronger all the time. Perform 5 sets of 15 repetitions with 60 seconds break between each set. Take 90 seconds after completing 5 sets.

Side Planks: 5 sets of 45 seconds each side. Start with the side plank on your left side holding for 45 seconds before going straight to your right side for another 45 second hold. Repeat for 5 sets off of each side with minimal rest.

Burpees: 4 sets of 30 seconds work, 30 seconds rest. Perform as many burpees as you can in 30 seconds followed by a 30 second break. Repeat for 4 sets.

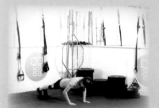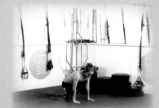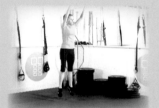

15 Minute 'Finisher': Next you will have another finisher, a little longer than Monday's. This is a tough one!
- 400 metre run
- 10 Push Ups
- 10 Hip Bridge

Find a running track or somewhere that you can mark off 400 metres. Start with a 400 metre walk, jog or run. Whatever you can manage looking to cover the 400 metres as quickly as possible. Next perform 10 push ups and finally 10 hip bridges. This is one round. Continue for 15 minutes completing as many rounds as possible in the allotted time!

Cool down!

* See recipe on page 103.
** See recipe on page 104.

Meal Plan

Breakfast: Scrambled eggs with turkey bacon, grilled tomatoes and mushrooms.

Snack: 100g full fat Greek style yogurt with a scoop of protein powder.

Lunch: *Quick and easy salmon cakes with green beans and steamed broccoli.

Dinner: **Chicken tandoori.

Snack: Tin of salmon.

DAY 18

DAY 18 WORKOUT:
5KM AND CORE!

Warm up.

Back to the session from day 11! Today, the goal is to cover that same 5km in less time than you did last week. Double check the time it took you to cover 5km before starting. It's much easier to beat your time when you have a number in mind (the power of goal setting). After you've completed the 5km take a 3-5 minute break before performing 5 sets of planks holding for 45-60 seconds each set with a 45 second break between sets.

Finish your session with a thoral stretch.

Meal Plan

Breakfast: Scrambled eggs with turkey bacon, grilled tomatoes and mushrooms.

Snack: Chicken breast

Lunch: Steak with steamed veggies.

Dinner: *Pat's paleo pizza.

Snack: 100g cottage cheese

Motivational Playlist as Suggested by the PDF Facebook Fans

1. **Groove Armada – Superstylin' (Gabriel & Dresden)**
2. **Beyonce – Crazy In Love**
3. **Britney Spears Ft. Will.I.Am – Scream & Shout**
4. **Fragma – Toca's Miracle**
5. **Benny Benassi – Satisfaction**
6. **DJ Fresh & Rita Ora – Hot Right Now**
7. **Awolnation – Burn it Down**
8. **Diplo – Boy Oh Boy!**
9. **Prodigy – Warriors Dance**
10. **Madonna – Hollywood**

* See recipe on page 104.

DAY 19 WORKOUT: 'THE GRADUATION WORKOUT'!

Warm up.

Squats: 5 sets of 20 repetitions. Perform 5 sets of 20 repetitions with 60 seconds' break between each set. Take 90 seconds after completing 5 sets.

Push Ups: 5 sets of 15 repetitions. Perform 5 sets of 15 repetitions with 45 seconds' break between sets. After your last set take a 60 second rest.

Burpees: 5 sets of 15 repetitions. Perform 15 burpees before taking a 45-60 second break. Repeat for 5 sets.

Planks: 5 sets of 1 minute holds. Perform 5 sets in the plank position looking to hold each set for 1 minute. Take 45-60 seconds' rest between sets.

20 Minute Finisher: Last one to finish! You've got a 20 minute finisher which will consist of completing as many rounds as you can of:
- 400 metre run
- 15 squats
- 10 push Ups
- 5 burpees

Cool down!

Meal Plan

Breakfast: Bell pepper stuffed with beef mince.

Snack: Half an avocado.

Lunch: *Spicy turkey meatballs.

Dinner: **Thai baked cod.

Snack: Carrots sticks with two tablespoons of homemade hummus.

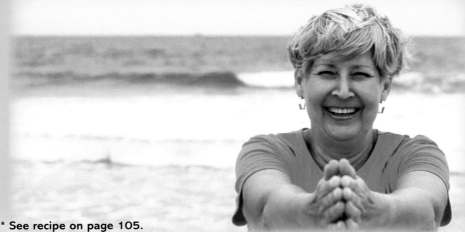

* See recipe on page 105.
** See recipe on page 105.

DAY 20

Meal Plan

Breakfast: *Rising Stars chocolate milk.

Snack: Small serving of cashew nuts (8-12).

Lunch: **Soup

Dinner: ***Garlic and lemon roast chicken.

Snack: Small handful of pumpkin or sesame seeds.

* See recipe on page 97.
** See recipe on page 100.
*** See recipe on page 106.

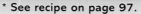

DAY 21

The results of your 21 days of hard work should definitely be noticeable by now. Look at how good you look and feel! You probably never thought you would get here but you have, so I truly hope that the past three weeks have shown you what your body is capable of.
Well done!

Meal Plan

Breakfast: Grain free porridge with scoop of whey.

Snack: Chicken breast

Lunch: Egg salad

Dinner: *Beef burgers in a lettuce wrap.

Snack: Hard boiled egg.

DAY 20/21:
ASSESSING YOUR PROGRESS

Take your measurements, and set new goals to help you continue your new lifestyle.

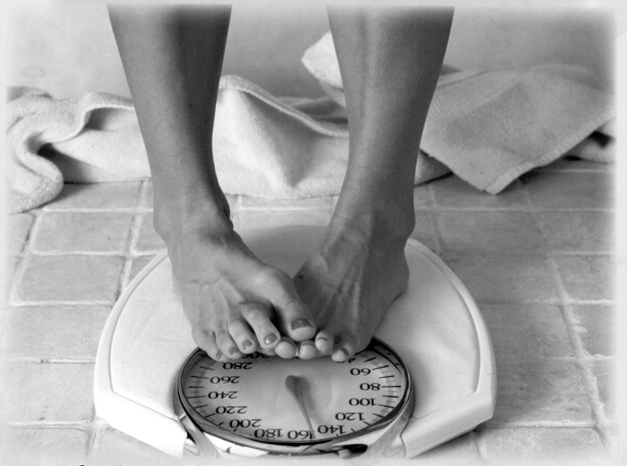

* See recipe on page 102.

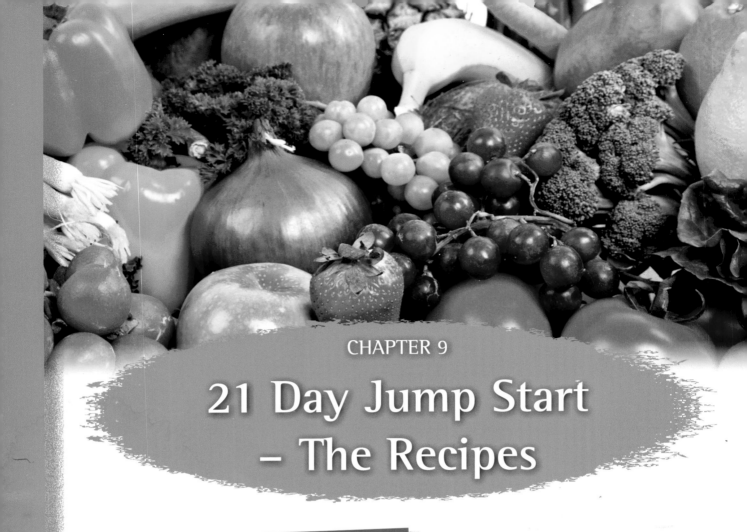

CHAPTER 9

21 Day Jump Start
– The Recipes

BREAKFASTS

Divilly's Berry Blast Smoothie

Ingredients
Handful of frozen blueberries
2-3 frozen spinach cubes
2 tablespoons of Greek style yogurt
1 scoop of whey protein powder (preferably strawberry flavoured)
1 tablespoon of coconut oil
Handful of ice cubes
1 cup of almond or coconut milk

Method
Add all ingredients and blend until fully mixed.

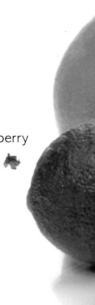

Rising Stars Chocolate Milk

Ingredients
1 cup of almond milk (unsweetened)
1 scoop of chocolate flavoured whey protein powder
1 tablespoon of almond nut butter
1 tablespoon cacao nibs
3 tablespoons Greek style yogurt
Handful of ice cubes

Method
Add all ingredients and blend until fully mixed.

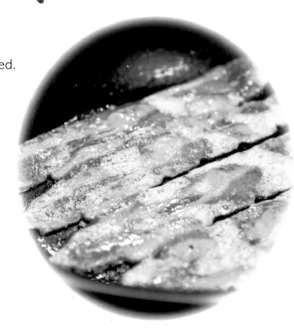

Silver Strand Pina Colada Smoothie

Ingredients
1 cup of frozen pineapple chunks
2 tablespoons of desiccated coconut
1 cup coconut milk
1 scoop of banana protein powder
1 cup of ice

Method
Add all ingredients and blend until fully mixed.

Healthy Full Irish

Ingredients
Gluten free sausages
Turkey rashers
2-3 scrambled eggs
Mushroom
Tomato
Coconut oil
Small sweet potato, peeled and grated
Onion
Garlic

Method
1. Add your grated sweet potato and onion to a small pan with a tablespoon of coconut oil. Mix in some crushed garlic and cook on a medium heat for ten minutes.
2. In a separate pan, cook your sausages, mushroom and turkey rashers, again with a tablespoon of coconut oil.
3. Cook your tomatoes on a low heat on a separate pan with the lid on. Once your meats are nearly ready, cook your scrambled eggs in coconut oil again and serve.

Bacon, Egg, Tomato and Avocado Salad

Ingredients
1 ripe avocado, chopped into pieces
2 boiled eggs, chopped into pieces
1 medium-sized tomato, chopped into pieces
2-4 cooked slices of bacon chopped into pieces
Salt and pepper to taste

Method
Mix all ingredients and serve.

SOUPS & SALADS

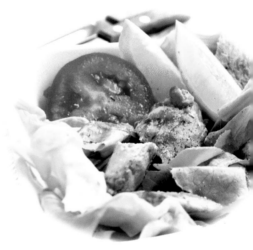

Muscle Builder Salad

Ingredients
Chicken breast (diced and marinated with paprika spices)
Mixed greens (spinach and rocket)
Tomatoes
Jalapenos
Sliced avocado
Toasted seeds

Method
Toss all ingredients together and add juice of half a lemon to dress.

37 West Superfood Salad

Ingredients
Mixed leaves, spinach and rocket
Beetroot
Broccoli
Quinoa
Feta chunks
Sun blush tomatoes
Toasted seeds

Method
Toss all ingredients together and add juice of half a lemon to dress.

Garlic and Red Pepper Cauliflower Hummus

Ingredients

2 cups of steamed cauliflower

2 tablespoons of almond nut butter

2 cloves of garlic

3 tablespoons extra virgin olive oil

Pinch of sea salt

Splash of lemon juice

Method

Add all ingredients to food processor and blend.

Galway Guacamole

Ingredients

3 avocados

Juice from 1 lime

1 small shallot, minced

3 generous pinches of sea salt

Freshly ground pepper

Method

1. Combine your minced shallot, salt, and lime juice and leave to sit for ten minutes.
2. After pitting and peeling your avocado, place half the flesh into a bowl and mash.
3. Pour the lime mixture into the same bowl to combine with the mashed avocado.
4. Dice the remainder of the avocado flesh into small cubes and incorporate into the mixture in the bowl.
5. Add freshly ground pepper to taste.

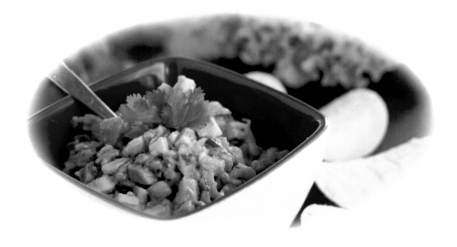

Tomato Soup

Ingredients

1 tablespoon extra-virgin olive oil
1 small onion, chopped
2 cups vegetable or chicken broth
1 can (400g) diced tomatoes
2 tablespoons tomato paste
1 teaspoon dried basil, crushed
1 cup of canned coconut milk
¼ cup fresh basil, chopped

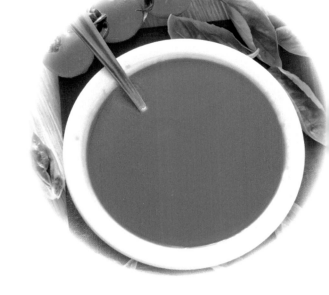

Method

1. Heat the oil in a large saucepan over medium heat. Add onion and stir occasionally, cooking until soft.
2. Add the broth, tomatoes, tomato paste and dried basil. Bring to the boil. Reduce to a low heat, cover and allow to simmer for around twenty minutes.
3. Leave to cool for ten minutes.
4. Add your mixture to food processor and mix until smooth.
5. Return to saucepan, add the coconut milk and cook until heated.
6. Garnish with fresh basil.

Broccoli Soup

Ingredients

500g broccoli
1 tablespoon of coconut oil
1 leek, sliced
1 rib celery, sliced
4 cups of chicken broth
2 cups of coconut milk
1½ tablespoons of coconut flour
1 teaspoon chopped fresh thyme or ½ teaspoon dried

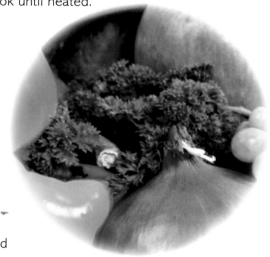

Method

1. Cut the broccoli into florets and put to one side.
2. Next chop the stems and set aside.
3. Trim and discard the tough, fibrous skin from the stems, coarsely chop the stems and set aside.
4. In a medium saucepan over a medium low heat, heat the oil, cook the leek and celery, stirring occasionally, for eight minutes, or until the leek is soft.
5. Add the broccoli stems and broth. Bring to the boil, then reduce to a low heat, cover and simmer for 15 minutes.
6. Add the broccoli florets and simmer for a further ten minutes. Transfer the mixture to a blender or food processor. Puree until smooth. Return to the saucepan and increase the heat to medium.

7. Meanwhile, in a small bowl, whisk together ¼ cup of the coconut milk and the coconut flour, until smooth. Slowly add to the broccoli mixture, stirring constantly. Stir in the remaining 1¾ cups coconut milk and the thyme. Cook, stirring for 3 minutes, or until thickened.

LUNCHES & DINNERS

AJ's Mexican Turkey Burgers

Ingredients
500g turkey mince
1 small onion, finely minced
1 garlic clove, finely minced
1 tablespoon chopped coriander
1 teaspoon paprika powder
1 teaspoon oregano
½ teaspoon cumin
1 tablespoon coconut oil
Salt and pepper to taste

Method
1. Mix the turkey mince, onion, garlic, coriander, paprika, oregano and cumin in a large bowl.
2. Leave to sit for 30 minutes in the fridge.
3. Add coconut oil to a pan on medium heat. Meanwhile, preheat your oven to 160°C.
4. Mould your turkey mixture into 4 even-sized 'burgers' and fry on the pan for around two minutes, turning them at the halfway point.
5. Transfer to the oven and cook for around 15 minutes or until cooked fully through.
6. Serve with a mixed salad.

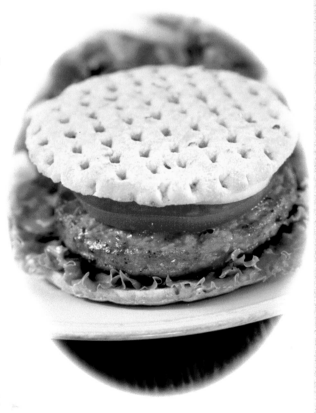

Barna Beef Burger

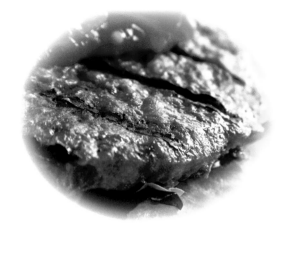

Ingredients

1kg beef mince

1 large onion, minced

1 clove of garlic, minced

¼ cup almond flour

2 eggs

½ tablespoon paprika powder

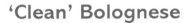Salt and pepper to taste

Coconut oil

Method

1. Pre-heat oven to 150°C.
2. Cook the onion and garlic in a pan with coconut oil until soft.
3. Mix all ingredients in a bowl (including onion and garlic).
4. Form into even-sized burgers and cook on a pan for around two minutes or until browned on both sides.
5. Transfer to oven and cook for a further 20-25 minutes or until cooked through.

'Clean' Bolognese

Ingredients

1 tablespoon extra-virgin olive oil

½ onion, finely diced

1 carrot, finely diced

2 celery stalks, finely diced

½ cup mushrooms, sliced

1 red bell pepper, thinly sliced

3-4 garlic cloves, peeled and finely chopped

500g of beef or turkey mince

Salt and pepper to taste

½ cup coconut milk

800g of canned tomato

¼ teaspoon crushed red pepper flakes

1 teaspoon oregano

1 teaspoon basil

1 teaspoon thyme

Coconut oil

Method

1. Heat a saucepan over low heat.
2. Add olive oil, onion, carrot, garlic, mushrooms, red bell pepper, and celery and sauté until lightly caramelised, (about 12 minutes).

3. Add beef or turkey and cook until browned, (about 10-15 minutes). Make sure to break up meat into small pieces! Drain off most of the fat and stir in 1 teaspoon of salt.
4. Deglaze the pan with a bit of water, stirring to loosen the browned bits on the bottom of the pan.
5. Cook for a couple of minutes, until water has evaporated. Add the tomatoes and stir in coconut milk, black pepper, red pepper flakes, and herbs. Gently simmer for 40 minutes, or until sauce has reduced and thickened.
6. When sauce has reduced, stir in 1-2 tablespoons of coconut oil and season to with salt and pepper to taste.

Salmon Cakes

Ingredients
1 large sweet potato cooked and mashed
$^1/_3$ cup almond flour
½ cup finely chopped parsley
2 tablespoons finely chopped onion
1 tablespoon fresh squeezed lemon juice
½ to 1 tablespoon hot sauce
½ tablespoon salt
1 teaspoon cumin
1¼ teaspoon paprika
½ teaspoon freshly ground black pepper
2 large eggs
2 cans of wild salmon
2 tablespoons organic coconut oil

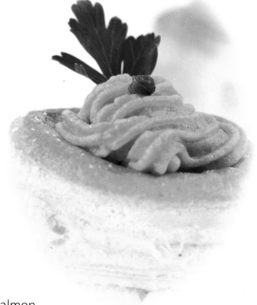

Method
1. Cook and mash your sweet potato and place in a large mixing bowl.
2. Add your almond flour, chopped parsley, onion, lemon juice, hot sauce, salt, cumin, paprika, black pepper and eggs.
3. Remove skin and bones from the canned salmon and crush into the mixing bowl with your hands.
4. Stir until well mixed then mould into fish cake 'patties' and place on a baking tray.
5. Heat a large pan and add coconut oil. Allow the pan to get very hot before adding your fish cakes.
6. Cook for 4 minutes each side and serve fish cakes hot!

Chicken Tandoori

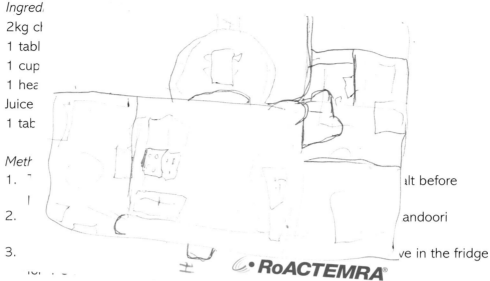

Ingred...
2kg cl...
1 tabl...
1 cup...
1 hea...
Juice...
1 tab...

Meth...
1. ... lt before
2. ... andoori
3. ... ve in the fridge
4. When ready to cook, preheat your oven to 180°C and ... or around 40 minutes, flipping the chicken at the halfway point.

Paleo Pizza

Ingredients
4 eggs
$1/3$ cup ground flax
$1/3$ cup coconut flour
½ cup milk (almond or coconut)
2 tablespoons spices (sea salt, garlic, basil etc.)
Goats cheese
Additional toppings

Method
1. Preheat oven to 180°C.
2. Place parchment paper on baking tray.
3. Mix dry ingredients and wet ingredients in separate bowls.
4. Mix all ingredients together and spread evenly onto parchment paper.
5. Bake for 10 minutes before flipping and baking for a further 10 minutes.
6. Add desired toppings to crust and then place back into the oven and bake until goats cheese is melted.

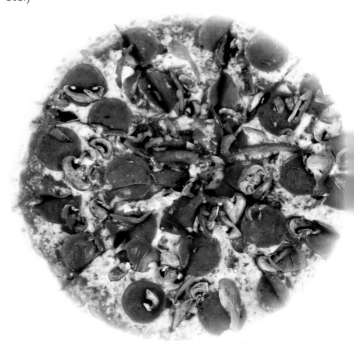

Spicy Turkey Meatballs

Ingredients

700g lean turkey mince
2 tablespoons garlic powder
½ tablespoon cayenne
½ tablespoon onion powder
½ tablespoon dried oregano
¼ cup chopped onion
¼ cup chopped red onion
½ tablespoon chilli flakes

Method

1. Preheat oven to 180°C.
2. Mix all ingredients in a bowl and form into meatballs.
3. Bake for 25 minutes.

Thai Baked Cod

Ingredients

4 cod fillets
3 stems lemongrass, chopped
2 red chillies, chopped
2 cloves garlic, chopped
Piece of ginger root, chopped
1 onion, chopped
1 lemon
4 tablespoons coconut oil
Salt and pepper to taste

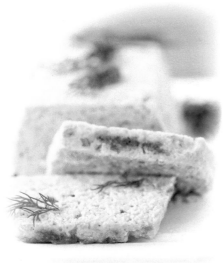

Method

1. Place your cod in tinfoil, and add salt and pepper to taste.
2. Slice half of the lemon and press the juice out of the other half.
3. Mix the ginger, lemongrass, lemon juice, chillies, garlic and onion and place mixture over your fish.
4. Drizzle the coconut oil on top. Wrap the foil over your fish and cook for around 25 minutes at 180°C.
5. Open the foil. Arrange the lemon slices on top and serve.

Garlic and Lemon Roast Chicken

Ingredients

¼ cup coconut oil

8 chicken thighs, with bones and skin

3 cups onions, sliced

3 cloves garlic, minced and smashed almost to a paste

½ cup lemon juice

2 extra lemons, thickly sliced (remove seeds)

1½ cups chicken stock

A bunch of picked thyme leaves

Sea salt and freshly ground black pepper to taste

Method

1. Preheat your oven to 180°C.
2. Melt half of your coconut oil in a large, hot pan and brown the chicken pieces on all sides.
3. After 5-6 minutes set the chicken aside.
4. Cook the onions until soft before adding your garlic.
5. Add the chicken stock, thyme and lemon juice and return the chicken thighs to the pan, skin side up.
6. Bring the contents of the pan to a simmer before covering and placing in oven for 20 minutes.
7. Remove the pan from the heat before adding your sliced lemon.
8. Return to bake for a further 15 to 20 minutes.

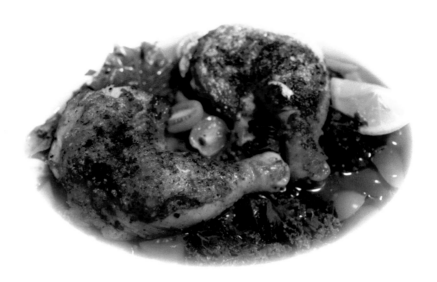

Mythbusting:
Five Health Foods That Aren't Healthy

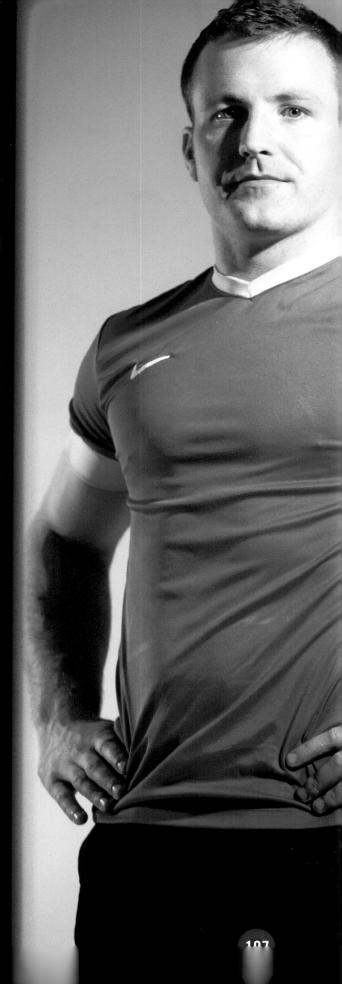

1. Energy Bars
High in 'empty' calories that are refined and processed. Sugar is the primary ingredient. The same goes for protein and meal replacement bars.

2. Fruit Smoothies
A lot of people have come to see fruit smoothies as being a healthy alternative to soft drinks. In reality, however, both shop-bought and home-made fruit smoothies are loaded with ridiculous amounts of sugar, which, except in the rare exception of a very active individual, will not be used, and consequently, stored as body fat.

3. Soya Products
Soya products have been marketed as a perfect protein source for vegetarians. It may, however, wreak hormonal havoc, particularly for men. It has also been linked to breast cancer, thyroid disorders and impaired fertility.

4. Wholegrain Breads and Pastas
These were made out to be a saviour in the battle of the bulge. They are slow-digesting sugars but still sugars! Also contain gluten.

5. Fast Food Salads
Dressings high in fat, sugar and calories. Can often make them as bad as the burgers and 'junk' food.

Fionnuala Baynes (Galway)

For me, PDF classes aren't about losing weight. I have always had a fair level of fitness and I love to try new activities. Before PDF I was bored of training alone all the time, and eager to make it more enjoyable. That was nearly a year ago now, and, in the meantime, I've completed my first half marathon... in 2:02! I never thought I could. What I've gained from Pat's classes is an overall level of fitness far beyond what I was managing on my own, even with cycling, running, horse riding and those monotonous gym sessions! To train for the half marathon, I supplemented classes with just one long run per week. That's pretty good going! Pat's nutritional advice has been key to my success to date. It's easy to get caught up with what foods are 'good' and 'bad' but now i just focus on what will make me feel better and improve my training. I feel stronger and fitter now than I ever have. I haven't reached all of my goals yet but with Pat's guidance and inspiration I can only go up from here!

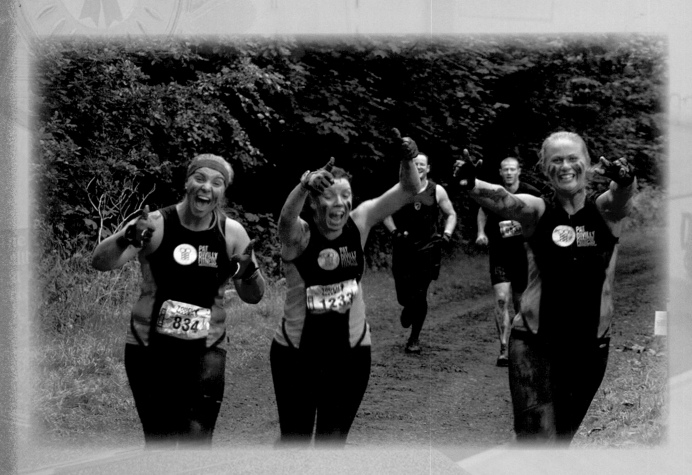

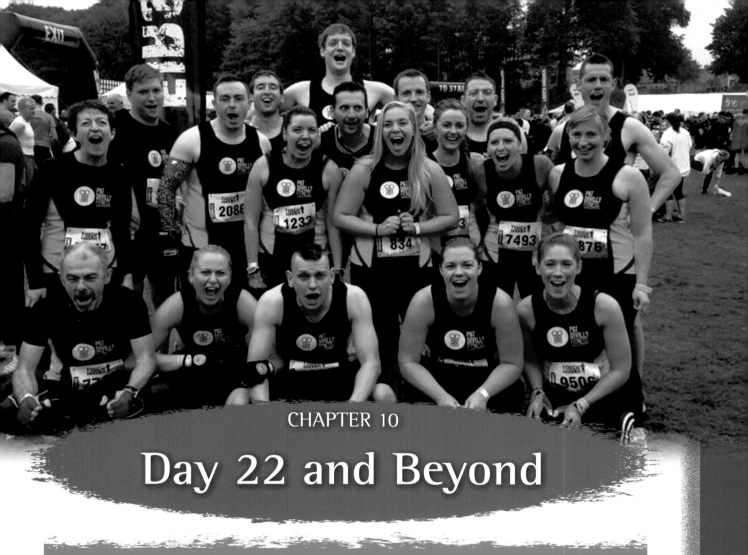

CHAPTER 10

Day 22 and Beyond

'I'm taking all the negatives in my life, and turning them into positives.' - PITBULL

Hopefully, the past three weeks will have changed your mindset and forced you to look at food from a different perspective. Ideally, you should see food as a fuel, and not a reward or a comfort. Similarly, you should see your training sessions as a productive form of self improvement, and not as a chore.

From now on, whenever you are about to eat, I want you to ask yourself if you are genuinely hungry or if you are trying to change your mood. Identifying the reason puts you in a position of power. When it comes to addressing issues in your life, look for alternatives to comfort eating.

The first 21 days were strict, but, rest assured, you don't have to live like a monk in order to continue reaping rewards from your new lifestyle. The plan set in motion the good habits you need, but now you are free to stretch the boundaries a little while still staying on track.

Remember, it takes 21 days to form a habit, and my *21 Day Jump Start* has simply prepared your body for a new life of healthy habits. You won't need to be as stringent with the nutrition, but you will know from the previous three weeks which foods worked best for you.

This isn't a diet, this is a lifestyle choice.

People will often recall a specific diet they carried out, and how they had lost so much weight with it at first but then piled it back on as soon as they came off the diet. Usually, they will blame the diet and say it's no good. Believe me, it's not the diet that is failing you! The reality is that when you start removing toxins from your system, your weight will fall. However, as soon as you start reintroducing those toxins back into your body again, the weight will inevitably return. This is why you need a new lifestyle, not a new diet. If nothing changes, then nothing changes! if you go back to way you used to eat, then your body will go back to the way it used to look. You don't need to be as strict with yourself from day 22 onwards. There will be room for cheat meals. In fact, I will be explaining later in this chapter how cheat meals can help your progress even more. See, it's okay to fall off the wagon every now and then, just don't set fire to it after you do!

> Carb cycling is the equivalent of an engine using more fuel on a long journey.

Carb Cycling

While a low carb approach will work for the 21 days, it won't work over a long period of time, so once you have completed the jump start plan, you should begin what's known as the carb cycling concept. On your more active days, increase your intake of gluten-free carbohydrates, such as sweet potatoes, vegetables, gluten-free porridge, etc. If your workouts take place Monday, Wednesday and Friday, then these are the days you need to carb cycle. You can take in these carbohydrates either at breakfast, or right after training, so as to replenish what you lost during the workout. Carb cycling is a really good option for people who are more active and want more variety.

The amount of carbohydrate you take in however, depends on how lean you are. If you have a lot of weight to lose, then you will not be taking in as much. If you are very lean however, you can afford to take in more. Likewise, if you are very active, it will be necessary for you to take in more. An endurance athlete, for instance, would have to take in a lot more carbohydrates, but you can be sure, they are eating good quality carbohydrates. The quality of the carbs is a massively important factor. Don't eat just any kind of crap.

> **Foods and drinks that claim to contain 'zero calories' are massively processed and not remotely natural. In fact, they are foreign to your body. They slow down your metabolism and mess up any chance you have of losing weight.**

Cheat Meals

When you are eating really clean, the cheat meals can actually be very beneficial to the weight loss process. They help fire up your metabolism again and your body is forced to quickly burn off the additional intake of food. Psychologically, cheat meals will also help keep you motivated.

If you have a lot of weight to lose, two stone or more, then maybe limit your cheat meals to once a fortnight. If you have more than a stone to lose, then you can have a cheat meal once a week. If you have less than half a stone, then two cheat meals a week are allowed. Everyone is different so just take this as a baseline.

Don't turn your cheat meal into a cheat day! Just choose a meal that you enjoy, eat slowly, and savour it. Don't gorge. You're not eating it for the sake of eating it, you're eating it because you want to enjoy it. It takes twenty minutes for your brain to register when your stomach is full, and this is precisely why it's important that you eat slowly. If you tend to eat fast, this is why you most likely feel crappy twenty minutes later.

A big mistake that a lot of people make is that they continue eating even when they are full. Once you feel full, stop eating!

When it comes to health and fitness, you can't fool nature; your body will tell you when you need to eat. If you are not hungry in the morning then you shouldn't eat breakfast. There is no point in force feeding yourself! It just doesn't make sense.

Cheat Meal Vs. Re-feed Meal
Integrate your cheat meal into your carb cycling. A cheat meal can also be a re-feed meal, which is basically a clean cheat meal. Where a 'cheat meal' will usually consist of bad carbohydrates, a 're-feed meal' will consist of good carbohydrates. Sweet potato fries would be a good example of a re-feed meal. A re-feed meal will fire up your metabolism in the same way a cheat meal would.

Pre- and Post-workout Nutrition

Play around with pre-workout nutrition. A general guideline would be to eat approximately one hour or 90 minutes before exercise. With the post-training nutrition, that twenty-minute window following your workout is when you need to eat some protein. You need to eat as soon as possible after your workout. (It's called the anabolic window, but let's be honest, a name like that would just put you off!)

Damage Control

Take Omega 3 fish oils, wheatgrass and glutamine before and after a drinking session! Glutamine will line your gut wall and take care of your stomach. Alcohol is massively acidic but wheatgrass will help alkalise the body.

If you are really craving something sugary, like chocolate, then the best time to have a square is right after your workout, literally within twenty minutes. (This doesn't apply to the plan for your 21 Day Jump Start! Day 22 onwards though, is fine!)

Training

Thanks to the 21 Day Jump Start, you now have great momentum on your side. You have built up a good base, you have become stronger and you know how to handle your own body weight. Maybe join a class, or sign up for a race. Constantly set performance-based goals. Stay away from the weighing scales. If you work towards a goal, such as a race, a goal that will improve your performance, then your weight loss and health will take care of themselves.

If you are working towards a race, you are less likely to eat rubbish. You are going to take better care of yourself.

Motivational Playlist as Suggested by the P.D.F Facebook Fans

1. Chase & Status – Hitz
2. The Bacon Brothers – Footloose
3. Rocky Soundtrack – Eye Of The Tiger
4. Freestylers – Push Up
5. For weight lifting: Skrillex with Kyoto
6. Korn – Coming Undone
7. Nina Simone – Sinnerman
8. Hardwell podcast 108
9. James Groarke – Tidal Wave
10. Wiz Khalifa – We Own It

Padraic McDonough (Galway)

Although I have been training with Pat for just six months, I have been following his nutritional advice and online training for the past year. In that time, I went from being a 14.5 stone couch potato, to an 11 stone active adult! I have superb energy levels which now make juggling life's responsibilities so much easier. Being self-employed and a dad of three kiddies, I often found that my energy levels were depleted, but, with training and nutritional expertise from Pat, I'm more active and energetic than I was 20 years ago when in my twenties! Above all else, I have enjoyed the journey and built it into my lifestyle. The energy levels in the group training are magnificent and we really help each other with our individual goals, all facilitated by Pat and his relaxed, yet driven, attitude. I have nothing but love, respect, and admiration for the man and his methods!

Marie Lavin (Galway)

To say that Pat Divilly has changed my life is an understatement. I first came across him in October 2012, when a good friend of mine did one of his programmes here in Galway. My friend is a slender size 10 and while I was impressed by the programme, and followed Pat's Facebook page with interest, I felt that at double my friend's weight, the PDF workouts were unmanageable for me. Typical excuse-

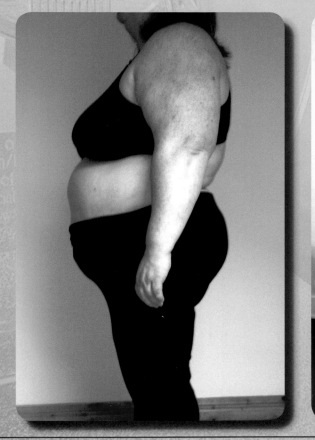
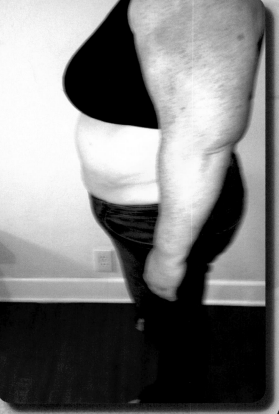

making syndrome! Fast forward seven months, and I finally took action. Pat's advert for his inaugural Six Week Summer Slimdown caught my eye, as it would finish the day before I travelled to the US for a family wedding, so I emailed Pat and told him about my concerns, that I wouldn't be able for the workouts. His response was that even if I followed just the nutritional guidelines I would look, feel, and move much better. He advised that I start slowly and incorporate the workouts gradually. I know this probably all makes perfect sense and doesn't seem like rocket science, but there was something in the way Pat spoke that struck a chord with me – no frills, no nonsense, do what you can, and you will achieve results.

And I did!

I followed his nutritional guidelines to the letter and am thoroughly enjoying eating good quality, real food. I concentrated on the food aspect for the first week, and then began walking the prom in Salthill every day in week two. By the end of week six, I had gone from 2km to 8km per day. On week three, I started to incorporate Pat's workouts. Even the warm up killed me at first but I'm getting there, very slowly! The weight didn't go on overnight and it will take time to lose, but, for the first time in a long, long, time, I feel that I am in control. On the six week programme, my weight dropped from 19stone 11bs to 17stone 13lbs, a total loss of 26lbs, almost 2 stone. While some of this would be fluid retention etc, I feel confident that this is the start of some dramatic changes in my life. I've lost 6 inches off my waist, from 54 to 48, 2 inches off my chest from 46 to 44 and 3 inches off my hips from 58 to 55. My BMI has also gone under 50 for the first time in years and my clothes, particularly my jeans and trousers, are falling off me! People have commented on my face, shoulders and waist looking smaller and I can certainly notice a big change in my midriff which was big both front and back. Pat was right. I am looking, feeling, and moving, so much better already! It's not easy sharing my measurements with anybody. They disgust me, and, to say I'm embarrassed, is an understatement. However, I am confident that my morbidly obese days are numbered. I'm well on my way to a healthier, happier me, and, if my story so far can help just one other person to get off their ass and make changes, then my mortification will have been worthwhile! I'm on holidays now in the US for a family wedding, not rigidly sticking to PDF, but incorporating what I can, when I can. My plan, when I get back to Galway, is to get right back on track and sign up to Pat's workout sessions in Barna. On the day before I left for my holiday, I declared out loud to a family member, 'this is not a diet, this is a lifestyle change', and then laughed out loud because FINALLY I understand! One last thing that should be said... while Pat can take full credit for transforming my attitude to food and exercise, the other members in the online group are superb. The support advice and encouragement is phenomenal. And PDF member number one is undoubtedly Magda. Her before and after pictures have inspired me beyond belief. As one of my friends said, 'Magda looks like someone who never had weight on' – the ultimate compliment!"

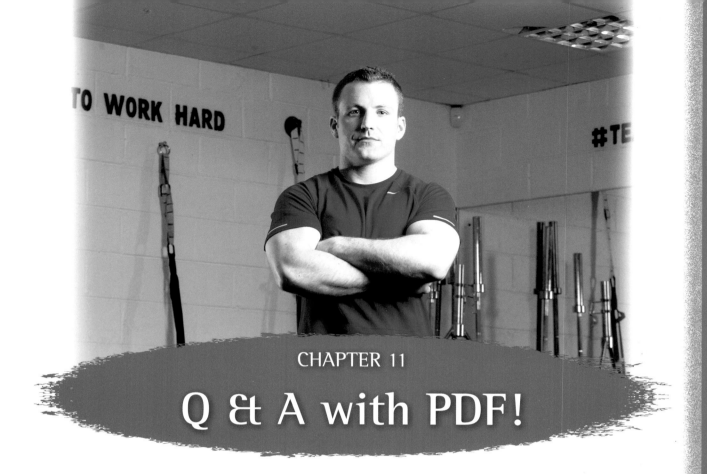

CHAPTER 11

Q & A with PDF!

In this section, I answer the top twelve questions I am most commonly asked on my 'Pat Divilly Fitness' Facebook page.

Q 1. Any tips on how to avoid giving in to temptation when I'm out shopping, or when I get a sugar craving?

Always eat before you go shopping. This prevent your hunger from encouraging you to take a walk through the sugar aisle! As I mentioned earlier in the book, a teaspoon of coconut oil right off the spoon is good for combating sugar cravings. The supplement, glutamine, is also particularly good for helping with cravings. The key to combating cravings in advance however, is to eat healthy fats with your meals so it suppresses your appetite and keeps you full for longer.

Q 2. What foods can I eat at night?

It goes back to preparation. Any of the snacks I have mentioned in the plan are fine. Healthy fats or protein would also be good if you are hungry at night. Forget that myth about not eating at night if you want to lose weight. You can eat at night, but only as long as the food you are eating is of good quality. For instance, gorging on carbs late at night will definitely hinder your weight loss process. (In fact, it's best not to eat carbs after 6pm) Some suggestions for evening/late night snacks would include cottage cheese, nut butters with sliced celery sticks, or some chicken. It's what you eat, that counts, not when you eat.

Q3. Are protein bars a healthy alternative to a chocolate bar?
No! They are full of sugar. If you want a healthy chocolate fix then have a square of good quality dark chocolate. This isn't allowed during your *21 Day Jump Start* however!

Q4. What nut butters are allowed in the plan?
Cashew butter or almond butter are the best. Organic peanut butter is ok, but cashew or almond are better options.

Q5. What is the best way to portion my meals?
A good guideline to follow would be a palm-sized serving of protein, a fist-sized serving of greens (have two if you feel like it), two teaspoons of fats such as nut butters or feta / goats cheese, or seeds, nuts or avocado.

Q6. How do I keep on track with my healthy eating, when I am raising children who won't eat the same foods as me?
With children, you have to teach them healthy habits. Stick with it and don't give in. If you are removing the junk from your own diet, why would you continue to feed it to your children? Their diet doesn't need to be as strict as yours, but similarly, it shouldn't be as bad as yours once was. Sugar is dangerously addictive and we are fed it from the time we are children. If you cut out the sugar from your kids' diet, then you are giving them a great start in life. Stand your ground and don't give in. They are putting up a fight because they think they can convince you to back down. They will resist this new food at first, but they'll eat it eventually if they are hungry.

Q7. Which is better? Tap water or bottled water?
Bottled water is better than tap water because tap water in Ireland contains fluoride which can consequently affect the thyroid. I am often asked about thyroid issues and the connection to weight gain. It is impossible to briefly tackle what is essentially a massive issue that no one has properly figured out yet. So many books have been written about this very topic and yet we still don't have a conclusive answer to it.

Q8. How can I lose weight when I'm naturally big boned?
You are not big boned. Your body wants you to be lean. When our grandparents were young, obesity was not a problem. There might have been one or two who were overweight, but obesity was not the issue that

it is today. It's not a medical or a genetic issue, it's about bad habits. Some people are less able to cope with sugar than others. There are plenty of people who can eat what they want and not put on weight, but you need to give yourself the best chance by following the right habits.

"I'm big boned" is an excuse. You're basically telling yourself that you will never be lean and healthy. Take responsibility for your weight, and suddenly you have a wealth of opportunities ahead of you.

Where you are now, is a direct result of the choices you have made to date, and everything you do going forward will either take you a step closer or a step further away from your goal. Using an excuse is not going to help you do anything productive, and if you are not being productive, you are not progressing.

Q9. What are the best foods to eat before and after a workout?

Your post workout meal is hugely important because it will replenish the body and help you reap the benefits of your workout. A whey protein shake is one of the best things you can take following a work out, because whey is digested quickly. It enters the bloodstream within twenty minutes. Glutamine is good for muscle recovery.

Q10. No matter how hard I try, I can't seem to shift the stomach weight. What am I doing wrong?

Check out the sleep and stress chapter for the most thorough answer to that question.

Q11. I drink a lot of caffeine, particularly tea. Should I come off it cold turkey, or should I wean myself off it gradually by switching to decaf for a while?

No. Do it cold turkey. Decaf drinks are not a healthier option. They are full of toxins.

Q12. Won't lifting weights make me look muscley?

Lifting weights will not make you bulky or stocky! Women just don't have the hormones to naturally pack on muscle in that proportion! Those female body builders you see are on steroids. Male body builders are eating at least six or seven times a day, as well as taking a massive amount of supplements, and then all but killing themselves in the gym, and even at that rate, it still takes a long time for them to pack on that muscle. Trust me, lifting a few weights won't make you muscley! If they did, then every lad would be walking around like Arnold Schwarzenegger.

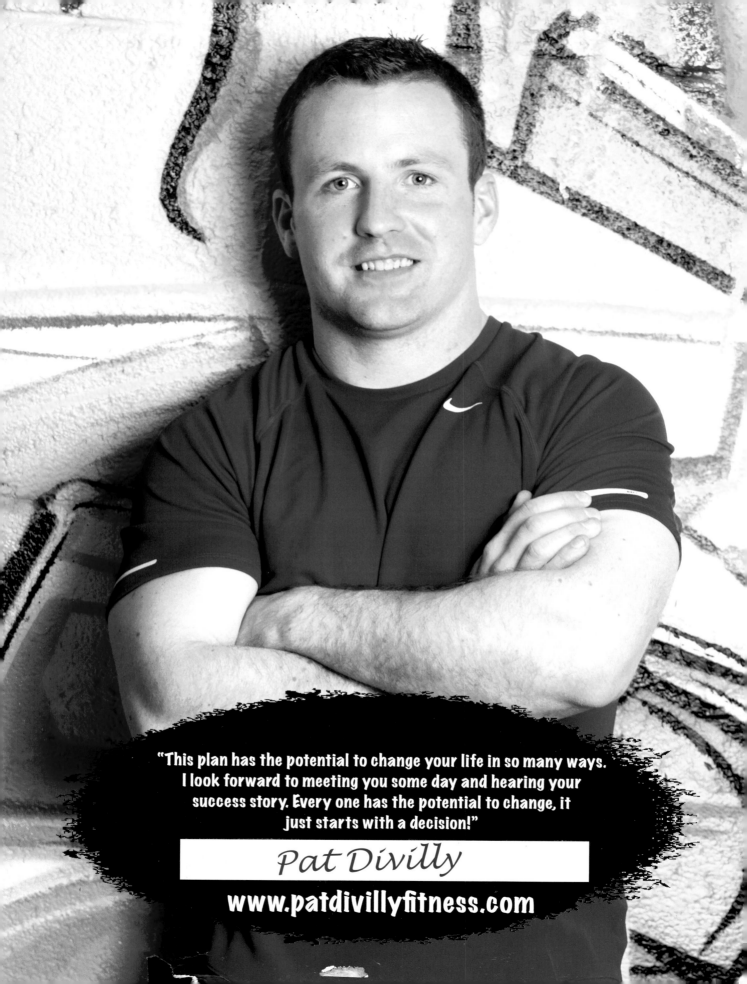

"This plan has the potential to change your life in so many ways. I look forward to meeting you some day and hearing your success story. Every one has the potential to change, it just starts with a decision!"

Pat Divilly

www.patdivillyfitness.com